Life Without a Bellybutton

Life Without a Bellybutton

Marion Barnes

Copyright © 2010 by Marion Barnes.

Library of Congress Control Number:		2010909732
ISBN:	Hardcover	978-1-4535-3161-7
	Softcover	978-1-4535-3160-0
	E-book	978-1-4535-3162-4

All rights reserved. No part of this book may be reproduced or transmitted in any form or by any means, electronic or mechanical, including photocopying, recording, or by any information storage and retrieval system, without permission in writing from the copyright owner.

This book was printed in the United States of America.

To order additional copies of this book, contact:
Xlibris Corporation
1-888-795-4274
www.Xlibris.com
Orders@Xlibris.com

Dedication

To my Mom for her unconditional love and inspiration.

To my husband for journeying through life
with me and creating a beautiful legacy.

To my talented daughter. Without her this book would not be possible.

Prologue

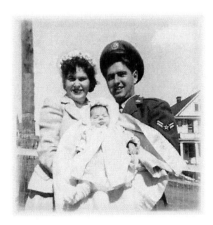

The nun whispered, "The baby has beautiful eyes dear, but we do not know if it is a boy or a girl."

The young mother acknowledges the sympathetic nun with a beautiful smile and replied, "I am starving. Could I have lunch please?"

The nun was eager to please the young mother and quickly replied, "Yes, Dear." After enjoying every morsel of her sandwich, the young mother was ready to face her new challenge, a name. With much wisdom, she chose Marion, an English name for a boy or girl. It was also her husband's grandmother's name.

My grand entrance into the world came with a good strong name, warm loving parents and undetermined sex. at the age of two, doctors did an exploratory surgery and determined I was a female.

The surgeries started at nine months of age. The reconstruction of my deformities was completed by age twelve. My medical records were like an interesting novel with a diagnosis stating multiple anomalies, including imperforate anus, separated symphysis pubis, and subcutaneous bladder in other words my back and pelvis were not connected and some of my organs were on the external part of my body. Nonetheless, Mom and Dad never reflected on my deformities and turned the focus on the fact that I had pretty eyes, a good name, and a warm and loving family.

Our family grew and Mom raised us in the Catholic Church. During one of my surgeries, a colostomy was to be performed; however, my colon miraculously became functional on its own. During the operation, I remember rising above the table and seeing a brilliant light. Out of the light, was a soft female voice that appeared to come from a woman draped in blue. She said, "It is not your time and you have a lot of work to do!" This memory is very special to me and I will never forget her and my special, spiritual experience.

The most difficult surgery I had to undergo was performed at the age of 6 ½ years old. I was taken to the operating room where a bilateral iliac osteotomies and bladder turn-in were performed. A body spike, also known as a cast was applied to my entire body.

The nuns at church told Mom not to spoil me, "Dear, raise her like you have six children!" My mother did end up having six children and strived toward not spoiling me. However, there were a few exceptions; for instance, Dad would give all the kids a swat on the bottom for misbehaving and when he got to me he swatted the side of the bed and told me to scream. Mom did swat me once when she realized I had shoved all my peas from a couple of weeks worth of peas down the chest of my body cast; I have to admit it was pretty disgusting.

By the time I was 7 years old, still unable to walk, doctors performed a surgery connecting my pelvic and back bone. The worst part of that surgery was waking up in a closed crib-like cage, scared to death and not being able to move. I was overjoyed to see Mom's beautiful cheery smile and her dark curly hair as she leaned over the top and peered in. She also assured me, "Everything is going to be fine!" Later I realized that she strongly and wisely held back her emotions from me.

I kept hammering questions at her, like, "Mommy, where are all those red things and parts of my body?" She acted like she did not know what I was talking about and continued to reassure me over and over again. My bladder was put back inside and I underwent plastic surgery. My back and hips were joined so I could walk correctly. Six months was a long time to be in a cast, but I survived.

Chapter 1

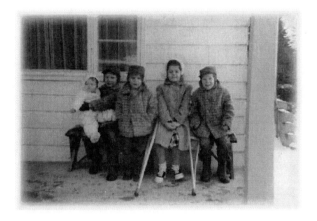

I recall back to when I was five years old, before I was in my body cast; Dad had received orders to go to Japan. I recall how hard they worked to get me released from Boston's Children's Hospital to travel. They succeeded and we went to Japan by ship. I am so amazed at how my mother faced each new challenge with enthusiasm and managed to make life so much fun. We moved outside of the base and lived in a Japanese neighborhood. Mom enjoyed adorning me in kimonos. My brothers and I rode giant turtles in the backyard. We loved to visit the Japanese candy shops right down the street. Attending school on base and being a kindergartener was challenging with crutches.

There was a boy in the school lunchroom that always smiled at me. He had gorgeous blue eyes but I never mustered up the courage to talk to him. Japan was also the birthplace of my first little sister, Patty. She looked quite different than I, with soft blond hair and pretty blue eyes.

After a year in Japan, we soon received a compassionate assignment at Otis Air Force Base on Cape Cod so I could be close to Boston Children's Hospital and Dad could continue with his Air Force career. Still in a body cast, I was never alienated from family outings. I remember how they would place me on a stretcher in the back of our wood sided station wagon so we could go to the beach.

Unable to attend public school in the fall, I started first grade with an awesome tutor that came to the house and a new baby sister. When winter approached, we were unable to attend the base Christmas program to see Santa. I could hear the disappointment in my younger sibling's voices and I knew it was my all fault; just as I was feeling down and guilty, the door bell rang unexpectedly.

My mother entered the room with tearful eyes, "Since we couldn't go to see Santa, look who came to see us!" We all squealed with glee when Santa appeared before our eyes in our own house! With Christmas being so special in the new base, naively, I shrieked joyously with delight. But, being a military family, staying in one place isn't the military life style.

After four exciting years in Cape Cod, from losing my body cast to being able to walk and go to a public school, Dad was reassigned to New York. Niagara Falls, NY was a short commute to Boston's Children's Hospital where I went for regular checkups. I always managed to keep my surgeries a secret as well as the fact that I did not have a bellybutton. I walked normally and appeared normal. But, Mom wisely prepared me for my next upcoming surgery.

During my twelfth year of life, I celebrated my seventh and final childhood surgery. The doctor, also a plastic surgeon, informed me, that this surgery will tighten up all the other surgeries to make me stronger; where, even though my bladder tuck was reinforced and plastic surgery on my abdomen was performed, I also presumed that I would get a new bellybutton. I do not recall any anxiety over the procedure at all. As a matter of fact, on my first day of recovery I had so much energy that I begged the nurses, "Please let me help you guys!" When Mom came into visit I was passing out meal trays with a big smile on my face. I eagerly introduced her to my new roommate, a princess from Saudi Arabia. I whispered to Mom, "She told me that birth defects are kept quiet or rather secret in her country." An awakening of my blessing became so revealed to me. I had realized how proud Mom and Dad were of me and how loving they were regardless of my defects. I was not hidden from the world like the Saudia Arabian princess.

It was time for the bandages to come off and expose a new me. In that unveiling moment, I was shocked with what I saw and cried out to the doctor, "Where is my bellybutton?" He replied in jest, "You do not want something that collects lint." In my mind, I was screaming, *Yes, I do!* And, life went on still without a bellybutton. I grew healthy and chubby as I entered puberty. Not having a bellybutton was quite an issue for me.

In that same twelfth year of my life, we remained in New York where I walked home from school every day in the frigid cold but never once complained as I appreciated the ability just to walk. I spent hours playing imaginary school with my sisters as they relished being the students and I the teacher in our old rented house.

My siblings and I had spent the summer with my grandmother, Mum Mum. We had enjoyed long days working in the garden and hanging clothes. She had six beds in the attic, one for each of us children. In the evening, Mum Mum would tuck everyone in but me. We had our special time with tea and cookies served on an artistically hand-painted plate as my reward for helping. By the end of summer, I was frantic when I realized I was 13 and weighed a hundred and forty pounds.

That summer, I had become deeply religious for such a young soul. I would often pray to God when I lit a candle at mass that God would let me have the holes in my hands that Christ had on the cross. In my young naive mind, it was a way of thanking him for my blessing and giving back as a purpose in my life. I pessimistically had thought my dreams of marriage and children would never be a reality, hence my prayer for purpose. However, with rowdy brothers, I couldn't stay too serious at mass because I had to interrupt their spitting contest from the balcony into the ladies' hats below.

Chapter 2

At age 13, Dad came home one evening and announced, "We are moving to Africa!" Preparing us so enthusiastically, Mom would proclaim, "We are ready for a new adventure!"

Before deployment in the fall, we planned a month long vacation at my parent's friend's summer house on the lake in New Hampshire. Dad and his buddy Pete would wake us up with the aroma of bacon and eggs. There was a long line in the morning to use the outhouse. On Labor Day weekend, we anticipated hot dogs on the beach. Trees surrounded the small lake with a tiny beach area and a wood raft a short distance in the water from the shoreline. I was slimming down and discovered I loved swimming. My hormones also started to kick in; even the song, "She Wore an Itsy Bitsy Teeny Yellow Polka Dot Bikini" bothered me because I knew I could not wear one because I did not have a bellybutton. I yelled at my brother, "They need to take that off the radio!" He just yelled back, "No way! It has a great beat!" I had thought the most fun of the vacation was swimming out to the raft and talking with Doris and Pete's kids, but little did I know, it could only get better!

Pete's son, Bobby, asked me to the end of summer dance. I ran and bragged to Mom, "Mom, Bobby asked me to the dance! Please can I go?" Pete overheard my pleas and insisted, "Yes, if you do your 'Wooly Bully' act tonight!" Wooly Bully was a popular song from the 60's and every time I finished a show, I would say "And Bully for You!" in my best Marilyn Monroe voice. That evening in front of the fire I sang off key to "Love Potion # 9." After that, Bobby and I were excused for our first date. We sauntered through the wooded area as the sun peaked through the trees.

At the dance, Bobby shyly informed me, "Marion, I do not know how to dance." I eagerly replied, "I dance with my family all the time and I watch American Bandstand. I will show you how!" We entered the rustic clubhouse building with hardwood floors and paneled walls.

Being the youngest kids there, we were both intimidated; that feeling quickly ended when the music started and it was "Do the Freddy." I squealed, "Bobby, this is easy! Raise your arm in the air and lift your legs one at a time." Sheepishly he replied, "Okay" and imitated me. We laughed and danced all night long. We even entered a twisting contest; even though we didn't win, people still admired our youthful gumption.

On the walk home, the wind kicked up and the trees danced as if anticipating the coming of fall, my favorite time of year. We could hear Mom and Dad still laughing around the camp fire, waiting up for us. I was shocked when Bobby quickly bent down and pecked my lips. We smiled and both headed home to share our great evening. I lay in bed awake for hours wondering why we had to move so far away? Even without a bellybutton, I had experienced my first kiss and lay awake in awe reliving every moment.

Libya in North Africa was different from any place I had ever known. Few families joined their military sponsor here but still base housing was full. Mom and Dad found a new villa to rent which was in a small town off the base for us to live in. It was high above the street that was lined with palm trees. The street was busy with Libyans riding camels and children briskly walking to school with books under their arms; you could see the women only revealing one eye while walking with woven bags of food. Young boys would drive by on bikes selling warm loaves of freshly baked bread. The villa was new and seemed quite cool with a strong scent of the stucco's wet plaster. The only washer machine mom could use was an old white ringer washer. She loved to go to the local market and get fresh fruit and vegetables, but everything had to be rinsed with a solution of bleach and water. Mom, with her positive attitude took everything in stride and even made shopping for vegetables fun. One day she took me shopping by myself. Mom declared, "Marion, you need a new bathing suit because there are beautiful beaches on base." We approached the gates of the base and there was a horrible stench. "What makes that horrible smell?" I asked as I wrinkled my nose in disgust. Mom pointed to the meat market where hooks hung with camel meat covered with flies. "Do people really eat that stuff?" Mom replied, "Of course they do, it is what they are used to. We eat cows!" We quickly escaped the smell by entering the Base Exchange to shop. Mom explained to me that I needed a bathing suit with cups in it now that I was developing. I chose a red one that really excited me. I felt so grown up. No one could see my scars or even know I did not have a bellybutton.

The base was off the Mediterranean shore. Swimming in the Mediterranean was amazing. The water was so clear and aquamarine in color. It was so warm compared to the Atlantic Ocean in Massachusetts. My brother, George, was my best friend there being that we were only eleven months apart. He had found a cove at the end of the beach where we could dive under and see amazing creatures and fish. Mom was so busy with the younger siblings she never realized how long we would disappear to dive. We had no fear.

Dad came home one evening and announced that our name had come up on the base housing waiting list. It would be safer for us to live there but we would only have two rooms. Mom said, "There is so much to do that it will not matter! We will set up three sets of bunk beds. We will make it work!"

The next day we were all busy packing. The neighbors had everyone to dinner but I stayed back to finish my packing. I was finishing up my room when the house boy entered and asked "Do you need help?"

"No I am just about done." I replied.

In broken English, he said "I can help like this." Instead of him helping to pack, he reached down and held my hand. I did not seem to mind at all until he pushed me on the bed so violently that I became so scared but was able to push him off and run to the neighbors. I never told a soul. Like all teenagers I yearned for romance, but I was aware of my emotions to know *that* was not romance.

Six kids in one room should have been a nightmare, but instead it was like camping out every night. School was an open air surrounded by palm trees. I even learned to play tennis.

I started babysitting and buying my own clothes. I was so proud when I bought my first mini skirt. "Mom isn't this so cute?!"

She looked me up and down, scowled and remarked, "It's a bit short isn't it?" But she never said I couldn't wear it. I felt so cool wearing it to school the next day.

At school, my homeroom teacher called me up front right away, "Marion you need to go to the office!" I was pretty shook up but prepared myself to hold my ground regardless of the issue. The principal came out of her office to approach me. She was a rather large woman in spiked heels and wore too much perfume. "Marion your skirt is too short, and I must suspend you the rest of the day. Do not return unless you are dressed appropriately!" I stormed out of the office and marched myself home to complain to Mom.

"I cannot believe she sent me home! How can she complain about my mini skirt when this is the 60's and so obviously in style? She wears too much perfume anyway! Doesn't she know it's hot here in Africa?!"

Quietly, Mom acknowledged, "Marion she is the principal and you must respect her." I was astonished that she was never angry at the fact I was suspended. At this point, I decided to get political. I had also previously purchased a green granny dress with a matching head scarf. They were just coming into style, too, and I knew its full length covered all my legs would be acceptable; I couldn't wait to challenge her. Feeling adorable, I entered homeroom only to hear once again, "Marion you need to go to the office."

The principal, again, approached me and said, "You are not dressed appropriately!"

This time I defensively stated, "But, my legs are covered!"

She wisely retorted, "You are different than others and will distract boys from learning." Even though I had learned a valuable lesson on the importance of not being a distraction, I still marched home in anger after being suspended once again. George agreed with me that it was not fair and so did Mom. I realized that my battle was not that important and returned to school looking like every other female student.

The school offered a trip for a fee of one hundred dollars to go to school on board a ship for two weeks for all those with good grades. I was thrilled that George and I had accomplished that.

"Man I want to go on that ship, but how would Mom and Dad afford to send both of us?" George questioned.

I somberly agreed, "They probably could not even afford to send just one of us." To this day I do not know how they did it but they surprised us and sent us both.

Mom and Dad took us to the port in Tripoli, the capital of Libya. We were looking for our ship the *"Davona."* George yelled "There it is, it's huge!" We had a teary farewell with our family and went on board. It was an amazing cruise ship all equipped with the crew dressed in white. Aroma of food came from the dining area. Our dorms had bunks supported by chains. *Lights out* meant time to sneak out the Ouija board. That stopped one night when we swore spirits made all our chains rattle! In retrospect, I am sure we just hit a big wave.

We attended classes and would stop at different ports along the Mediterranean. When we docked in Cairo all of us loaded buses and went to lunch along the famous Nile River. We sat at tables on a cobblestone area alongside the river. The ship had made us bag lunches to go on each stop. Students and teachers reloaded buses and headed to the Sphinx and Pyramids. We first toured the museum. I could not believe all the gold and artifacts from the tombs. We paraded to the Sphinx. There, stood camels and herders to take us to the pyramids. The camels hissed and seemed so scary. I flagged George down, "Look at me, I am wearing a short a-line dress and stockings. How do you expect me to climb up a camel?"

"Marion you will be fine, besides your dress is brown so it won't get dirty. It's the only way down to the pyramids, you can do it!" Then he proceeded to help me get on that nasty, hissing camel. I held on tight with my skirt riding up. With each step the camel took I slowly moved up and down. I gradually crept toward the pyramids when I heard a loud, booming laughter and, *Hello,* from my brother, George, as he trotted quickly past me riding on a horse leading all of his buddies. For some time, I never found that humorous. But the pyramids helped me to heal from my humiliating experience with their fascinating wonder.

Luckily, we were able to board buses without a camel ride! The sun was high over the edge of the desert with only a couple of hours until sunset. It was a marvel I knew I might never experience again. The farther we traveled away from them, the pyramids and sphinx now looked like a post card but I became acutely aware of their real existence. I sat on the bus quietly, pondering how I never wanted to forget that I witnessed one of the greatest wonders of the world.

Next stop was Lebanon and we shopped at "Gold City" which was a place in Lebanon with rows of jewelry stores and gold heirlooms. I bought a ring that had a snake dancing on it. One of the girls exclaimed, "That is ugly!"

I snapped back "It will be a treasure that will help me remember this forever!" The shop keeper then mounted a pearl on my 'ugly ring' that made it beautiful.

The island of Crete was next. We went through a villa-like building with artistically colored and crafted mosaics on several walls. It was so peaceful and lovely.

From there it was onto Greece where the itinerary showed a special dinner and belly dancers after shopping. However, it did not happen that way. One of the girls from our dorm had stolen some jewelry.

I was a loner and clueless of who did it. The Greek police interrogated our whole group of girls by questioning us one by one. I was so scared when one officer shined a light right in my face and yelled, "You know who did this don't you?"

Terrified, I answered, "No, Sir."

Yet, silently, I thought in my mind, even if I did know I would not tell because I would be too scared of what would have happened to her.

Again, he questioned, "Did you do it?"

I awkwardly replied, "No." However, I thought to myself, I was aware that one of the girls was a trouble maker and her parents had even fought for her to go on the trip.

Finally, he dismissed me to the hall to wait for others to be interrogated. We all whispered that we suspected we knew who the girl was that stole because for the rest of the trip she had assigned seating at the front of the bus next to the teacher. And, she was that trouble maker.

The remainder of the trip was quite difficult because I became dreadfully ill. Once I returned, mom took me to the doctor and I had developed pneumonia. I was so happy and relieved that I was home and could recuperate.

A short time passed and news of a political uprising spread over the base; Kaddafi, the Libyan leader, wanted the Americans out of Libya. Immediately, the water pipes were cut off that went into the base housing. My father was instrumental in setting up tents for families living off base. When we couldn't go to school I realized that this was a serious crisis. One morning we woke to thunderous explosions. Rebels threw hand grenades over the base fences. The command came down that all dependents were to be immediately evacuated to Ramstien Air Force Base, Germany.

It was so scary to board the plane without Dad. Mom's eyes were full of tears but she remarkably put on a happy face and constantly reassured us. I can't fathom how she must have felt moving on without Dad; leaving him in such a dangerous environment had to be more than worrisome. "Okay guys we are ready for another adventure and Dad will join us soon." She announced.

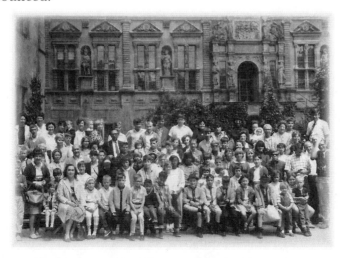

June 6, 1967: Evacuee from Libya, Wheelus Air Force Base, Germany, touring the Hidleburg Castle.

Chapter 3

In comparison to the dry desert sands of Africa, Germany was so green and beautiful. We were placed in empty military barracks. My younger sisters and brothers loved the long hallways to run through. We had our meals in the chow hall which was the same cafeteria that the soldiers ate in. Mom did make it an adventure and took us places around the base. My favorite was a fabulous maze cut out of bushes.

After one of those long fun days I asked my mother a question. "When is Dad coming home?"

"He will come home when Tripoli Air Force base is completely shut down." She quietly responded.

"Mom, where will we live?"

"Well, then we will get orders to some place safe, don't worry. I just received some checks, so tomorrow you need to help me buy everyone a winter coat. It will get a lot colder than Africa ever was."

"Sure Mom," I promised. Before we knew it, Dad had received orders to Hahn, Air Force Base in Germany, I was happy we did not have to travel far.

I fell in love with Germany. The base was small but had beautifully old trees everywhere.

It reminded me of New England. There was a long road that led to the housing area which encompassed numerous apartment buildings. Our apartment was on the third floor. It was large and Mom quickly made it home. Unfortunately, the laundry had to be done in the basement, not an easy task for a family of eight, but easier than using the old ringer washer in Africa. Our first meal was spaghetti and meatballs, a tradition each time we moved or celebrated something special. Dad would always say to Mom, "I love spaghetti and meatballs, but I love you more." Then he would break out in a chorus of songs like, "*A Your Adorable, B Your so Beautiful,*" and Mom would join with a romantic look in her eyes and using the wrong words attempted to harmonize with him. Dad would then rinse and stack all the plates for my mother to wash. They always seemed to work in harmony.

We were all settled in and it was time to start school. We rode buses to the main base and school. I was shy but usually blended in quite well to be unnoticed. Third period was over and a quirky, fun, red-headed girl said, "Hi are you ready for the real fun now?"

"What do you mean?"

"We have to load the buses for gym class and get our hair messed up from the showers!"

My heart started to pound in a panic because I would have to expose my scars. I followed the red-headed girl on to the bus in a fog. My mind was racing with thoughts of fear. Everyone will stare at my scars. They will laugh at me not having a bellybutton. The red-headed girl asked, "Are you okay?"

Awkwardly, I whispered, "I hate gym!"

"Me too! Lets skip."

I proceeded to add, "Plus, I don't have a bellybutton."

Unsure of this plan but petrified of showering I went along with it.

"My name is Doris, what's yours?"

"Marion," I responded.

Doris directed, "As soon as the kids line up, run to the back of the bus and sit on the floor."

"What about the bus driver?" I inquired.

"He always walks for coffee," she explained.

We followed her plan and succeeded. Then, Doris hit me with the first degree, "Why don't you have a bellybutton?"

I answered with details, "I was born with multiple birth defects, and my bladder was on the outside of my body. I couldn't walk until they put me in a cast all the way up to my neck. I was in it for six months. There were a lot of surgeries."

Doris looked at me with sympathetic eyes and then with a quirky grin replied "*Cool!*"

She then quickly asked with a teenage giggle, "Do you like G.I. S?" I was overjoyed that her sympathy was not going to rule our friendship and she was actually treating me like a normal teenager.

"Well Doris, My dad is a G.I."

"No, I mean young soldiers like Airmen. There are so many cute ones here on the base!"

"Oh!" I recognized. "I think they are too old for us."

Doris proclaimed with enthusiasm, "Some are 18 and 19 years old."

"Cool, but I am a little scared to date, remember I don't have a bellybutton!"

"Marion you're cute, they won't be able to tell." I broke into laughter and started to share her enthusiasm. Just then the class returned to the bus and we sat up in our seats. Our plan for avoiding gym class went on for days.

We quickly discovered that we lived just a few streets away from each other. We both had large families. Doris was so easy to talk to and I did not feel different than others. We schemed to go bowling on base and have fun with the intent to meet young G.I. s. In my eyes, life was good, until we got caught skipping. We both had detention, and served our time. From that incident, I gained the confidence with Doris by my side to talk to the gym teacher about my physical condition. I was able to skip showers. The first day on the gym floor was the beginning of basketball. When the time came to pick teams, I knew no one would want me because I could not run well. The girls came out of the lockers and gathered around. Somehow I found the courage to blurt out, "Okay girls I do not want to make any team lose. I can't run worth a darn. You could pick me on your team to be nice but deep inside you would hate me, but I would be a cute team captain! I am surely not the cheerleader type!" They burst into laughter and I became the team captain. I discovered a tool to help me cope with not having a bellybutton, a sense of humor!

I think Mom and Dad were thrilled with my new social life. I knew I was. They were preparing to go to Fascine, which is a celebration much like Mardi Gras. Mom came out of her room with feathers in her hair and fish net stockings laced up her legs. I could only imagine what Dad was wearing. Suddenly, a big sunflower peeked around the corner and sprayed my face with water! Holding the sun flower was a hilarious clown.

"Dad you do not match Mom!" I yelled, laughing hysterically.

"Now I know where I get my sense of humor from," I proclaimed proudly.

"Mom, I wish I had your legs!"

Mom smiled and said briskly, "Leave tomorrow night open, the neighbors downstairs have their French relatives visiting and invited you to join us for a seven course meal."

"Cool, have fun." I loved using my new expression.

I really wanted to go bowling with Doris but I moseyed down to the neighbors. Their apartment displayed wall to wall plants and hanging flower baskets. Birds in antique cages sang beautiful melodies. The table was set meticulously with white linen and wine glasses on each setting. Our host called everyone to the table.

From the hall, a handsome young man entered. "Everyone, I would like you to meet my nephew Jean and my niece Gisele. Gisele quickly smiled and said "Hello," with a thick French accent. She was tall, thin and so pretty with jet black shoulder length hair and pale skin. She spoke broken English and from school I remember broken French. Jean spoke no English but was quick to laugh and enjoy all the conversations. Their aunt served many courses of fabulous food. With each course, came a different wine or liquor that she insisted I tasted. Mom and Dad reluctantly allowed me a slight indulgence but after a few courses everyone was too happy to worry about anything.

My nose went numb so I stopped indulging but all the adults and Gisele went to bed. Jean pointed at the record player and I nodded yes and pointed one finger up as to say one minute. He nodded in return with understanding. I ran upstairs and entered our apartment. Quickly I tip toed into George's room and got some cool records. Then I ran to the bathroom to freshen up before running downstairs. Jean took the Steppenwolf album and played it. We both started to dance with enthusiasm. *Jumping Jack Flash* was a hit as well as *Born to be Wild* but he had other music to play. It was romantic, soft and sung in French. He whispered my name in a thick French accent and pulled me close to him swaying to the music. His cologne smelled wonderful and his face was soft and smooth. I closed my eyes and treasured the affection. He started to passionately kiss me, over and over again. I whispered "*Bonsoir*" into his ear and he echoed back, "*Bonsoir.*" I closed my eyes and thanked God for such a wonderful evening. I knew that may never happen again because he did not know that I didn't have a bellybutton and I had so many scars. I was glad he was leaving back to France tomorrow but I will hold the memory of that long, passionate kiss forever.

Mom called the recreation center on base and found out there was a bus leaving for Amsterdam. Gisele had stayed behind with her aunt a little longer. "Gisele is seventeen and wants to travel while here. Would you like to go with her?"

"Sure, that would be a blast!" I replied enthusiastically. Mom and her aunt made arrangements for a youth guest house that would serve continental breakfast and guide us in activities and events. We left for the weekend. The ride took us through Luxemburg and was so lovely with flowers and cottages everywhere. Luxemburg captured our attention as it was so clean and so picturesque. We pointed out things to each other but with her broken English and my little bit of French we mostly smiled and created our own sign language. Checking into our rooms went smoothly.

Gisele and I were both ready to go site seeing and venture out, but the hostile insisted we visited the cheese factory first. It was interesting but very stinky. Finally, we got to be on our own. We were told to be back by 10:00 pm. We nodded with no problem or contest. As we wandered away we pointed at the bridge to remember our way back to our room.

The daylight left leaving the night an adventure. The pubs seemed to all have welcome mats on the door, even for teenagers. Gisele spoke and laughed in French to everyone. People bought us food and drinks and the music played. We knew it was time to venture home and we found an American gentleman of whom I asked directions.

I proudly declared, "We are staying next to the bridge, could you please give us directions to our hotel?"

The man burst into laughter and replied comically, "Girls," he smiled, "there are over 400 bridges in Amsterdam!"

Feeling quite silly I thanked him and scrambled away. "Gisele we should have been better students," I blurted out as we both agreed and giggled! We went around the corner and saw all these windows lit up with women standing in them with price tags. I heard someone whisper that it was the red light district. We started to walk faster and somehow before dawn we did find our room in time for a continental breakfast and boarding of the bus. I realized on the way back that I liked growing up and knew this was not what a typical American teenager would be doing on the weekend. I was going to miss Gisele when she returns to France but I couldn't wait to tell Doris about the trip.

School would be out soon and summer would be in the air. Doris and I babysat and went bowling. I volunteered at the Red Cross to stay busy all summer.

Outside the base, a carnival was set up with a beer tent and band. Doris begged, "Come on Marion it will be a blast, let's go!"

"Okay, if my parents let me." Mom and Dad gave me permission as long as I was home by dark. Doris showed me an amazing path through the woods that led right to the festival. We had to watch for tree stumps but it was so pretty with all the tall old trees. We could hear the German music blasting through the woods before we left the path. It was quite festive. The band had on authentic old German attire; beer glasses were being raised underneath the big tents. The aroma of grilled bratwurst was everywhere. The carnival rides were right outside of the tents. "Let's ride on something fun!" Doris squealed. Then she rambled, "Look at all the cool guys here!"

"Most of them are G.I.s, they are not going to be interested in us, we are too young!" I quietly interjected.

Doris quickly came back stating, "Well I am interested in them."

I smoothly avoided the subject by changing it, "I am not too cool about scary rides, but I do love the merry-go-round." So, on the merry-go-round we went. It was a big step up for me to maneuver as I stretched my leg up a handsome young guy jumped in front of me and boosted me up." Thank you," I meekly said. Quickly, I scurried to a bench where Doris could sit beside me but instead she sat right in front of me. The young guy hovered over the bench and asked, "May I sit with you?" I could feel my cheeks flush as I nodded yes. He had a buddy that sat beside Doris. They quickly seemed engrossed in each other.

"I am Alan Schaefer from Bakersfield, California."

I liked his warm brown eyes and continued the conversation, "I am Marion Woods, and my Dad is stationed at Hahn Air Force Base."

Alan eagerly shared that he was a private in the army and he built bridges and did construction. I told him I had five brothers and sisters. He said he was 19 and I told him I was almost 16. (It sounded older than saying I was 15.) I did not realize that we had remained on the merry-go-round through several stops. "We better get off!" Alan said. He jumped off and then reached up and lifted me to the ground. Butterflies danced in my stomach.

I looked up and said, "Thank you sir, you are such a gentleman! It was so nice talking to you!"

Alan, not wanting to be dismissed so soon, replied, "Would you like to walk around together?"

"Sure!" I replied, a little too eagerly, "But let me check with my girlfriend."

After finding her in the beer tent, I whispered to her, "Doris, Alan wants to walk around together!"

"Cool. I will hang out with his buddy." I was happy she didn't want to walk with us. Alan and I drifted away and he reached down and held my hand. The butterflies bounced back.

We were so absorbed by each other I hadn't realized the sun was starting to set. "Oh no, I have to be home before dark! I need to go find Doris." We found her sitting in the tent with a group of Alan's soldier friends. I yelled over the music, "It's almost dark out we have to go!" She smiled a flirtatious smile and said goodbye to the handsome soldiers.

We started to walk quickly when Alan asked, "Will you be here tomorrow, umm, I mean would you like to meet me here at noon for a date?" I felt nervous about meeting him alone so I responded that I may have to take my sisters and babysit them. I loved taking my sisters places, they were so adorable and they helped make me feel secure. "That's great. It's a date then." He squeezed my hand as he grinned from ear to ear. I felt like Cinderella running home after the ball.

Doris jealously questioned, "How did you get the cute guy? I can't believe you have a date!"

"Me neither!"

"Are you going?"

"I am, but I am going to bring my little sisters, he said he didn't care. I have butterflies Doris, it's my first date! He doesn't know I don't have a bellybutton. He may never ask me out again!"

"Are you going to tell him?"

"Maybe sometime but I want to see what he is like, first."

The path was getting darker and now it was scary so we walked faster. I ran up the stairs to tell Mom I was sorry for being late. I excitedly recounted to her my exciting day. "Mom this guy, Alan, asked me on a date tomorrow! Can I go? I told him I had to bring my sisters." I received both their blessings and was told that I did not have to bring my sisters but at the end of our date I needed to bring him home to meet them.

I spent all morning deciding on what to wear. It was a beautiful day with a little cool breeze. I finally dressed myself in a floral knee length dress with a lavender rain coat. I had butterflies in my stomach again and such a wonderful feeling of excitement. Mom dropped me off at the festival grounds and there he was looking handsome in khakis and a dress shirt tucked in and his hair slicked down.

"Hi Marion, I was afraid you would not show! Would you like to walk to the base and see a movie?"

"Sure I love to go to the movies!" Alan reached down and held my hand again and we started walking. The butterflies were still there but I felt comfortable. I noticed every flower and every bird singing. The walk seemed so short and we chatted the whole time. The movie still had another hour before the doors opened so Alan suggested we sit on the lawn by a tall tree. I slipped my jacket off and sat on it.

Alan said so seriously, "You are so sweet. All the guys said I was crazy to date a dependent. They are just jealous. Most sergeants won't let their daughters see G.I.s."

"Dad said he wants to meet you if I date you again. Maybe after the movies you can walk home with me."

Alan seemed to get pale as he responded, "That makes me so nervous are you sure they want to meet an army guy? I have heard all kinds of stories . . ."

"Dad is not like that you will see, okay?" I interrupted. The theatre was filling up as we entered. I could not tell you anything about the movie. All I remember was how he caressed my hand the entire show.

On our endeavor back, "Come on Alan I will show you the path through the woods to the housing area!" I coaxed him.

"Marion I am not sure about this."

"Alan it will be fine, I promise, besides, I am not supposed to date until I am sixteen! If Mom and Dad like you as much as I do I will still be able to see you."

"Show me the way, I am putting my future in your hands," he replied.

I found the path and we slowly walked through the thick wooded area. The sun had started to set and it was getting dark. "Look!" I yelled, "There is the end of the path, I see the housing area lights!" Alan whispered, "Let's stop for a minute." He reached down and gently leaned his head toward my face and kissed me. I tingled from head to toe. The kiss stopped so abruptly and Alan scowled while straightening back up. "Oh my God, my pants just ripped! I can't meet your parents with ripped pants!" I burst into laughter and he was quick to join me. I assured him no one would notice because our house was so busy and loud. We walked up the three flights of steps to our residence. Mom and Dad were extremely cordial and my little brother Johnny was quick to sing, "Marion and Alan sitting in a tree, K-I-S-S-I-N-G!"

Mom even invited him to dinner the following weekend and I could see Alan's face break into a genuine smile. We exchanged phone numbers and our goodnights in front of 7 pairs of eyes.

When I lay my head down on my pillow that night, I went over the whole weekend relishing every moment and pondering how I would ever make it to the weekend. Then I gave thanks to God for letting me have a boyfriend even though I did not have a bellybutton.

I thought the week would never come to an end. Alan came to dinner and of course it was far from quiet. Everyone seemed to talk at once. The chatter all stopped when my brother Johnny accusingly blurted out, "Marion has a hicky!" Defensively, I shouted. "I do not!" I could see Alan's face blush and he seemed very uncomfortable.

Dinner was finally over and the conversation had turned into a more than pleasant direction. I could not wait to walk Alan to the end of the housing area.

"Mom, I am going to walk Alan out and we are going by Doris's quarters first," I stated while trying to make our escape. Mom replied that she needed Alan to help her in the kitchen first and asked me to go brush my sister's hair. It seemed to be an eternity before we left.

Alan held my hand and we went into the hallway. He whispered, "I thought we would never be alone."

"Me too!" I whispered back, "Follow me." I led him to the eves of the apartment quarters. "Let's move past our unit, we can make this our secret place." We found a comfortable spot and sat down. It wasn't long before we embraced each other and began kissing passionately, like I had never done before. Alan stopped abruptly and began to talk, "Marion we should not be this close. In the kitchen your Mom told me about all your surgeries. I am so sorry. She said I had to be a perfect gentleman and respect you and be gentle. You are so sweet and it is hard to be this close to you."

"Don't feel sorry for me, I am perfectly fine now, I love being close to you. Kiss me a little longer and then we will go," I pleaded. He walked by himself out of the housing area to make up for our time in our secret place. I could hardly sleep wondering if he would be too nervous to see me again. I knew I did not want sympathy. Should I have told him I didn't have a bellybutton? He probably will never call again. All I could think about was why Mom had to tell him all that stuff about me. I made up my mind not to confront her, though.

All my fears drifted away when Alan called and invited me to a picnic with all of his buddies the next day. I was so proud to be at his side. Every guy was eager to talk as well as tease me, all in good fun. All of them insisted on walking me home. When we arrived, I could not believe how cool Mom was when she invited them all up for chocolate chip cookies. As they were leaving she invited them the following weekend for bratwursts.

It was an amazing time. A time I hoped would never end. It was a starlit evening and Alan took me into the baseball field. We laid down in the dugout, out of site from anyone. Alan held me so tight and then he started to sob quietly. "Marion, I have orders."

My eyes welled up with tears as I babbled, "When and where?"

Alan's voice became soothing when he replied, "This is so hard because I love you. We are being deployed in a few weeks to Vietnam."

I shivered and could not comprehend the sadness that had overwhelmed me. I didn't follow the news much, but everyone knew how many young men had died there.

"Marion, we will spend all the time we can together. Some of my friends are not going and I will have them watch over you," he reassured me.

I cried all the way home.

The following week was full of life changing events. Dad had orders, too, for Warner Robins Air Force Base in Georgia. I knew they wanted the East Coast because it was close to Boston, Massachusetts, I do not think they were happy with the south, though. Mom, as usual, was quick to adapt and start a new adventure. I recognized if Alan remained in Germany, moving would have been devastating. Alan's visits were further apart with them preparing to leave.

Doris called and said, "Alan told my boyfriend to tell you 'good-bye' because he could not do it himself. He loves you and they are leaving today. Let's walk to the base and see them caravan out." It was too sad to understand not saying good-bye so I dried up my tears and somberly walked to the base with Doris. Sure enough, all the army vehicles were lined up by the field. My tears started to roll again. "Doris I think I need to go home!"

Dust started to fill the air as the vehicles were lining up. Suddenly, a jeep did a sharp u-turn and was heading in our direction. Doris screeched, "I think it is heading towards us!" The jeep was heading toward us so quickly that dust and dirt was flying in its trail. All the guys look alike in uniform but my heart skipped a beat when Alan jumped out. He ran and squeezed me so tightly. "Marion, all the guys said not to say good-bye personally but I could not do it! I love you! You will have a wonderful life. I just know you will have four kids and a station wagon!" He finished his embrace and speech with a long tearful kiss. I was happy and sad and promised, "I will wait for you and we can write!" He jumped in his jeep and disappeared in the dust into a convoy of unrecognizable faces. All I knew is he loved me and this was the saddest thing I had ever felt.

Life was hectic preparing to leave Germany. Mom and I did tons of laundry to prepare to pack up. I was grateful to go to bed tired so I did not have to think. Leaving Germany was tough but like Mom I was ready for a new adventure. I walked to Doris's house for the last time. "Man, how am I going to stand not being able to see you and talk to you everyday?" I whined.

"Marion, we will be in touch. You have my address and phone number, I know you can't afford to call overseas but we will be back to the States next year." She broke into tears and we hugged good bye. We both knew it would never be the same.

Chapter 4

The travel time to Georgia was exceptionally long and once we arrived, it was not what I had expected. We were all cramped into temporary housing. My new experience with humidity was hard to embrace especially when I caught glances of my frizzy hair staring back at me with a mind of its own from the mirror. The sweat poured down my neck as I complained, "Mom it is so hot, where are we going to live?" She replied, "Dad just called and said there is no base housing available for three months! Tonight we are going to check out a trailer park." Dad ended up finding a long silver Airstream trailer and refurbished it by stripping it and adding three sets of bunk beds. We moved out of temporary housing on Warner Robins Air Force Base into a trailer at a trailer park in Perry, Georgia.

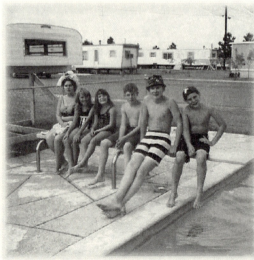

The park was eye appealing. In the center of the parked campers was a huge swimming pool. Mom said surprised, "Even though you have to start back to school, we are on vacation for three months!" Dad parked our camper next to a picnic table and we all jumped in the pool. The next day seemed like a real vacation. Mom said we need to enjoy the day and then it is off to enroll in school. I knew I was advanced in French so I was very excited about French class. It was quite a shock when a boy came up to me in his deep southern accent and very slowly, slaughtering French asked me, "Par . . . lay . . . vous . . . france,,,, saaaay?" It took everything I had to keep from laughing so I gently nodded my head and replied "Oui" and looked away. Lunch time was there before I knew. The sun shined so nicely and I sat out on the hilly front school lawn under a tree. The hilarious boy from French class joined me. "Can I Sit here?" He asked in his southern brawl.

"Sure, but do not speak French!" I yelled.

"Where are you from with you accent?"

I responded, "My family is from Boston and my dad is military, we just arrived from Germany and we are staying in the trailer park until we get housing."

He replied, "Soooo cool." Then he rambled on and on, "My dad is the town mortician. That is what I want to be when I grow up. We should go on a date and you could come to our morgue. We can be there right when a body arrives that is the best time. Some times they sit right up and you get scared to death, like they are really alive!" That did it for me, I burst into laughter. "Okay we can hang out but no morgue for me!" "Fine" he quickly responded. Then he battered me with a series of questions about places I had been, "Man you must have lived all kinds of places, tell me, where do they talk different, how long does it take to get to these places?" Saved by the bell, I was relieved to go back to class.

My favorite time of the year was always fall with the cooling temperatures and the colorful leaves, but in Georgia it seemed more like summer. My naturally curly hair did not like the humidity no matter what season. I didn't complain too much because the constant warm weather graced us long enough so we could swim after school and Dad would come home and light the grill.

Mom burst into laughter when I shared the story of my new mortician buddy. I was thrilled to finally meet a nice girlfriend, Debbie. We quickly became close friends and she was eager to invite me to her home. Her beautiful southern home sat away from the highway surrounded by acres of land.

Dad asked, "What time should I pick you up tomorrow?"

"After lunch, we will be sleeping in after staying up so late."

"Okay, see ya later alligator," he waved as he drove away. Debbie's parents seemed older than mine but quite friendly and extremely hospitable. They had a house full of guests all talking in such a thick southern accent it was difficult to decipher all their conversations. We joined her mom and sat on the front porch over looking some magnolias and peach trees. Her mom said, "I reckon it's getting cold. I think I will go in."

Of course that is not what I heard; actually, I had never even heard the word *reckon*.

I quietly whispered to Debbie, "What's wrong with your Mom's rectum, is she all right?"

Debbie confused inquired "Why do you ask?"

"Well I thought she said her rectum was cold so she went in. It certainly isn't cold outside—well compared to Germany, and I had rectum problems at birth."

Debbie headed in her Mom's direction and repeated what I had just said. In less than a minute the house was echoing with laughter. Debbie's dad said I was welcome back anytime and they were going to teach and educate me all about the South. I told Debbie I was so happy to have found a best friend as well as a second family.

Every day I checked the mail with great expectations of a letter from Alan, only to be disappointed. We were finally moving into base housing where I hoped his letters would find me easier once we were there. Setting up the house and decorating was so much fun, that I would fantasize doing my own house with Alan one day. We lived in the trailer for so long all the space was fabulous. I did miss all the swimming and grilling though. I started a new high school, Warner Robins High. On day one I knew I did not belong. I came home in tears. "Mom it was awful there. I could not believe the football players push kids out of the way. They fly the rebel flag and nobody talks to the Negro kids. I just hate it!" Mom comforted me but said, "Your job is to get an education and learn about different environments. Prejudice is something you have never known it is a horrible thing but it does exist.

In the weeks and months to come, I worked hard to get good grades. I loved art and enjoyed that class. Our project was to select a partner and create a collage. The Negro girl beside me did not have a partner and we did ours together. When we finished she shyly looked at me and said, "It's good but I sure hope you don't get in trouble." I looked around at our classmates projects and thought we had out done all of them. We walked up to the teacher's desk and placed it on her desk. With great anticipation we returned the next day wondering what our grades would be. We received an "F." In shock, I approached the teacher and defensively asked why we received an "F." She disgustedly gazed at my partner and said, "You know why you failed!" In disbelief, I left not understanding this thing called prejudice! I informed Mom of the incident ands she was on the phone with the principle and had our grades overturned. I was so upset!! The white maids were called by their last name and the black maids were called by their first name. I did not want Mom to handle this one so I planned a sit in. Of coarse I was sent home and Mom did find out anyway. My brother George did start a Rock Band and that helped me find a way in by being his groupie! I made a new best friend "Karen"! I knew she at first just wanted to hang around my brother and his band but we became buddies even away from the band! We had moved off base in to a real house. We all loved it and George's room was in the garage where he could also have band practice. I was finishing up my junior year when we heard that our house was rezoned for a different high school. I was actually excited to attend North Side. I would still come home to our cute rancher house and check the mail to hear something from Alan.

Unexpectedly one evening I received a call from Doris, "Hi Marion, how are you?

I was so excited to hear her voice, "Wow! I am doing great, what's up with you?"

"I just got a call from my buddy in Alan's unit and I am so sorry and she burst into tears blubbering he wanted me to tell you Alan was killed." A great feeling of sorrow fell over me and tears rolled down my cheeks."

"Doris, are you sure?"

"Ya, I am so sorry."

"Doris, how would I find his family? All I know is that he is from Bakersfield California."

"I don't know. I will ask if he calls again okay?"

"Okay." With one phone call my life had changed. I cried in Mom's arms and she comforted me and we tried with no avail to locate information on Alan. I cried myself to sleep every night for three months and I became angry about the war.

I enjoyed my friendship with Karen. She included me with her large family of six kids and I with my large family of six kids. We both loved kids and our families. She was determined to marry Richard, her brother's best friend, and was quite confident she would. I loved her simple nature and her smile. She had beautiful, long, blonde straight hair that I would have given anything for because I had to iron my hair and roll it into orange juice cans for straightening. She was an angel at a time that I really needed one.

Debbie had met a soldier and stayed pretty busy with him; it was hard to be around her because it reminded me of Alan. She always wanted to be a writer and I only hoped she would follow her dreams.

Mom wanted me to be more active and did not approve of my hatred of the Vietnam War. One evening she said to me, "Marion, instead of being angry why don't you do something about it, like join the USO?" Her suggestion struck a nerve and I decided to visit before school started up.

I was very nervous when I entered the USO building. I was greeted with such enthusiasm and given a tour. They informed me that I could not be married or engaged and I had to give all the soldiers equal attention. I left there an official USO girl. It felt good and I could not wait for the first meeting and getting involved. It brought tears to my eyes seeing all the soldiers standing around. It seemed like their home away from home.

My senior year started, hurray! I only had to attend a half day so I joined DECCA which is a school program that allowed us to work and get credit for it while going to school. I worked at the local hospital as part of my business class credit. Making friends at the new school was so much easier. Everyone in the DECCA class had good grades. There were a lot of military dependents as well. My first friend was a tall redhead named Barbara she was smart and fun. Barbara introduced me to a short brunette named Renee who introduced me to Rhonda. Rhonda had a boyfriend that was going to Vietnam. Rhonda and I also worked at the hospital together. We were partners for everything, the only problem was that she passed out at the sight of blood. I covered up for her all the time.

On school break we were all together and I decided to invite them to the USO, "Hey guys tonight I am going to the USO, do you want to join me?" Rhonda said her boyfriend would not like it but she would go when he leaves. Barbara loved the idea so of course Renee wanted to try it too because those two were joined at the hip. That evening they attended and they all became USO girl volunteers. A few times a week, we attended dances, played games, put on floor shows and served themed dinners like taco night or beenies and weenies to the troops. Every time I heard a soldier was going to Vietnam I planted a kiss good-bye on his lips. The girls teasingly called me *Hot Lips Houlihan* from the hit TV show, MASH. I could not let any soldier leave feeling unloved. The USO kept my mind and heart healthy. I would go to class, then go to the hospital and then straight to the USO. The girls talked me into going on base to an airmen's dance. I loved dancing so it sounded fun. We were being silly, laughing and dancing with each other when a man in tight jeans and a white shirt approached me and said he loved my legs and asked me to sit with him. "Hi, I am Ralph and I would like to take you out sometime. I am in the Air Force and I have my own car, unlike a lot of these guys." "Okay Ralph, here is my phone number, call me. You will have to meet my folks first though." I gathered the girls and we jumped in the car. I bragged that Ralph asked me out and I gave him my phone number. "He didn't sweep me off my feet but it would be so much fun to have a boyfriend for the holidays!" The next day Ralph called. We planned a date for Friday night. He drove to the house in a beautiful red Camaro. I introduced him to Mom and Dad and we headed out. He took me to a dark restaurant and talked all about himself. After eating we sat in the bar where he abruptly said, "I can't believe you haven't noticed my muscles, I am a weight lifter.

"Oh." I said sipping my ginger ale, "My brothers will be impressed."

"Would you like to see them?"

"No I believe you. We should leave soon I have to work the hospital tomorrow."

The next day when I got off work I entered the house to see a dozen roses on the table. You would have thought they were for Mom with all her excitement. On the card read: *Marion I want to see you again, love Ralph.* Mom questioned the lack of enthusiasm I displayed. "Marion if you are happy seeing someone you should be excited." I replied confused, "I guess I am but I have a lot to do." I spent the evening at the USO. I really loved being there. It made me feel like I was making a difference. I told the girls about Ralph's roses. They too were so excited and cooed, "How romantic!"

Every weekend I would spend one evening with Ralph the other at the USO. I was grateful that he never seemed to mind me going there. The holidays came and went. I was so excited to turn eighteen. I could legally drink but it was not my thing. Ralph only seemed interested in me having sex now that I was 18 and I tried to avoid that too. One gloomy weekend in February he came over to take me to the movies. Instead we went parking and he proposed, "Marion, I have orders to Italy. Let's get married."

"Sure," I replied with indifference due to his lack of romance and the lack of chemistry. But, getting married is all I ever wanted, and he was excited enough for both of us. All night long I thought how if I was planning this with Alan I would be so overjoyed but I kept reminding myself that I couldn't put myself through that emotional torture.

We continued on planning our special day in March. Mom seemed a little reluctant but stayed busy planning also. Dad was proud I was marrying a military man. I went to a boutique to pick out my dress with my friends.

"Oh my that is the one!" The girls echoed from the bridal party. I glazed in the mirror and began to laugh. "I look like a southern bell!" It stuck out like a colonial ball gown and completely overtook my 5'2" 113 pound body. I shrugged my shoulders and settled for the gown. It was late and all I wanted to do was get in my robe and relax. The house was quiet except for Mom and Dad talking in the backroom. They hung a curtain that you could pull for privacy but it was left partially opened. They did not hear me come in. I peeked in at them to say *hi*, but I chose not to interrupt. Dad had opened a bottle of champagne and they were toasting. As their glasses clicked, Dad said, "Marion's medical bill through CHAMPUS is paid in full!" Tears rolled down my cheeks, I could not believe they were still paying medical bills from all my surgeries as a child. "Helen, I will find a way to pay for the wedding too," were the next words spoken to the next toast. My heart filled with joy and love toward them. I tip-toed to my room, not wanting to disrupt the moment.

The following week Ralph took me to the Base Exchange to buy a wedding ring. I was excited to have a ring to show off and be proud of. We went to the jewelry counter where I loudly proclaimed that we are getting married.

Ralph quickly interrupted rather abruptly, "Could you please just show us some rings!" His sharp words killed my enthusiasm immediately.

He snapped, "Which one do you want?"

I ignored his mood when I saw all the glittery jewels. "There are too many choices but I love the shiny wedding band, what do you think?"

He retorted, "I don't care just pick one and let's get out of here." My stomach was tied in knots and doubts started to fill my mind. But I just couldn't start to have doubts now that all the arrangements were being made. My aunt and uncle were flying in, Mom and Dad reserved the club and the cake was ordered. I just put it in the back of my mind and asked God to make things all right. Mom was pretty good reading my mind so I entered the house as cheerful as possible to show her the ring. She calmly acknowledged it and said it was quite beautiful; suddenly, shocking words came flowing from her mouth, "Marion I think with the wedding only a week away Ralph should move in here so we can get things done together." Astonished, I replied, "I guess it would be easier."

The next day he moved his things in while I was at school and work. I was so annoyed when I found a pile of his dirty uniforms on the floor cluttering my little room abandoned there, waiting for me to wash them. Also, left in the family room where he was staying, were a number of wedding gifts from his family that were in unwrapped boxes as if he had opened them without me. I found Mom sitting at the table eating a whole bag of peanut clusters, rather attacking them.

"Mom is everything okay?"

"I can't believe your fiancé put this bag of candy in the refrigerator in a house of six kids with a sign on it reading 'DO NOT EAT THEY ARE MINE.' He has some nerve. I am glad he is going to be your husband and not mine."

"Mom he is probably not use to a big family. What is with all these gifts opened?"

"Marion I think this is from a previous wedding, the boxes are dusty. Why don't you call his mom?"

"I will meet them at the wedding." We went through the boxes and I did not want to admit to my mother that the stuff looked old. Once again I put these thoughts too in the back of my mind.

Dad had the rest of the week off and I was excited I was going to fix both of my favorite men breakfast. Being the oldest of six I had become quite a good cook. Mom and the guys sat at the kitchen table and I served scrambled eggs, bacon and toast. Dad was thrilled with his breakfast but Ralph shoved his plate on the table rudely remarking, "I can't eat a cold breakfast." Mom left the table to busy herself and I offered to warm it up for him but he left abruptly to go out to the base. Mom and Dad were out doing errands when I heard a scream in the garage. My little brother Kenny had joking tried to compare muscles with Ralph and Ralph punched him in the stomach. I comforted Kenny. "Ralph that is uncalled for!" I was so angry and it was only two hours until the wedding rehearsal! Ralph apathetically called out, "Anyway, I am leaving now to meet up with my best men. Marion I will meet you at the church, don't worry Kenny will get over it." Mom and Dad came home from the airport with Uncle Tommy and Aunt Bonnie. Everyone was filled with wedding joy and excitement even Kenny. Off to the church we went. Ralph and his buddies were standing outside laughing; only one of them I recognized. I waved at Ralph and he waved and then turned his back to talk with his buddies. I felt so distant from him and sad. I wondered why he didn't introduce me.

Finally, he walked over and started a conversation. "Marion I will go to school before we go to Italy but I don't want you to drive my Camaro, I am going to put it up on blocks. Also . . ."

The priest interrupted him by calling everyone into the church to begin practice. We had chosen a ceremony where we walked down the isle together after the bridal party. We began our march when all my doubts overcame me and I whispered to him this doesn't feel right are you sure you want to do this? He angrily through his arms up in the air and said, "What's wrong with you?" While he finished the walk to the priest, I ran into Daddy's arms crying. I lifted my head to see Mom making the sign of the cross and mouth the words *Thank You God*! It hit me like a brick when I realized how in her unique wisdom, Mom having Ralph stay with us would reveal what a marriage would be like with him. I heard Ralph plead, "Give us a minute and we will proceed." The wise priest said humbly, "When doubt has been shown I can not marry you for another six months." Surprisingly, Ralph cried and continued to apologize. He came home and got his things and called his parents. His mother asked to speak to me, "Don't worry dear this happened the last time when he wanted to marry someone else that's why we didn't send presents." I went with him to the barracks to help him unload and say good-bye. He came back in the car and said we should have talked a long time ago. He was supposed to get married last year and never talked to the girl and she had broken it off too.

"Ralph you have been so rude and mean," I explained.

"But Marion, I really love you and want to marry you—maybe we can try again in six months?" He looked down and then continued, "I have to admit, though, I was a little hesitant about marrying you, too, which might be why I've been a little rude, I mean, you have a great figure and legs but with sex being so important to me, I was scared of how it would be with all your birth defects and scars . . . I mean, you don't even have a bellybutton. What if you can't satisfy me the way I like?"

There I was, an emotional wreck with a horrible migraine which I never had before, so that night in the car, I had sex with him. It was fast and meaningless. I just wanted to prove that I could be normal even without a bellybutton.

He drove me home and did not come in. I went straight to my room feeling ashamed at what I had done but I did realize I did not love Ralph and would never marry him even though I knew he wanted reconciliation. I made up my mind to go to nursing school and to have no more serious relationships, for a long time. That night I prayed to God to forgive me and thanked him for showing me the way. I told him all I wanted was a family and a man to love me for the way I am. My head hurt so badly but that night God became my best friend and confidant.

Chapter 5

The wedding day became the *unwedding* day. Mom seemed to take great joy in removing Ralph's name off the cake. Everyone was invited over later for the *unwedding* party. Mom and Dad made the best of everything and were ready for life to move on. I still felt remorse about last night but I also wanted life to move past this. That afternoon, before the party, I went to hang out at the USO for a while.

My buddy, Jim, was hanging out there and was so surprised to see me. "Marion I thought you would be on your honeymoon by now?"

"No I could not go through with it. I am the marrying kind but I didn't realize what a jerk the guy was!"

"That's okay now you can plan on marrying me one day!"

"No wedding for me Jim." I said laughing, "But speaking of weddings do you want to come to my unwedding party later?"

"Man your parents are so cool, I'll be there!"

The party went well with lots of laughter and sympathetic smiles. My head still throbbed but I survived. I think I dreaded even more going back to school unmarried and being whispered about.

The following day Jim called to take me to dinner. He was such a nice looking guy with a slight built and dark smooth hair, Dinner was perfect at a fancy steak house with candles on each table.

"Marion you are so sweet. Ralph is a fool to have let you go. I love your looks and how you take care of yourself."

"He kept rattling on about only wanting two kids. In the back of my mind, I could only think of my family tree and knew I would not always be a seven junior petite and I wanted a house full of kids! Well, Jim, dinner is so wonderful but I need to go home my headache has returned."

Jim drove me home and I went and hid in my bedroom with the lights out because the headache was so bad. The pain was so intense that my mother had to take me to the emergency room. I didn't have to face school the next day but my headaches did stop with the medication. Tuesday I went back to school where all my friends were wonderful and compassionate. I was even glad to be back at the hospital the following weekend to work. Life returned to normal and Mom warned me not to bring another guy home for at least six months. I was more than eager to oblige, "No problem Mom! A month had passed and with April right around the corner, I was looking forward to graduation. I spent most of my free time at the USO, which is where I was headed to that night. I quickly asked Mom if I could use the car but my brother George had already gotten permission to use it. Mom ordered him to drop me off and pick me up at nine o'clock. He was a little annoyed being my chauffer.

"You always get the car, I didn't want to share it tonight, not even give you a ride," he complained.

"George, I am older."

"Only by 11 months and we were born in the same year! Anyway, I am glad you helped me get the gig at the USO. We are playing next week, so thanks."

"Cool you know all my girlfriends will be there. If I didn't know better I'd swear that they like you more than me!"

He smiled like he already knew, "Well, bye Sista!"

"Don't forget to pick me up!"

I loved entering at the USO. The big sign over the parking lot made me feel patriotic and the club had become my home away from home. All my friends that I helped recruit would gather in front of the glass office window. "Hurry up Marion, the newspaper guy will be here any minute." The director of the USO was so proud to be awarding us our 200 hour pin. I felt pretty important having my picture in the paper. When the picture was done we opened the door that entered into the game room and cafeteria. We had served beanies and weenies. I whispered to Rhonda, "This isn't my favorite thing to do. I cannot wait for next week when my brother George's band is playing." Rhonda was much taller than I and heavier with long, curly, sandy blonde hair. We both worked at the hospital together, she was confident that she would be an R.N. even though she passed out at the sight of blood. I had introduced her to the USO because her boyfriend had just left for Vietnam. I wanted to make the time pass easier for her, I was always overly concerned with the soldiers after what had happened to Alan and I wanted her guy to hurry home. We manned the serving line for all the guys to come and eat. A cute young guy came through the line first. He had sandy brown, curly hair with the most amazing blue eyes that I had to tilt my head up to look into because he was so tall. He asked for extra beanies and weenies and of course he got it. After Rhonda served his rolls she could not stop babbling how cute and polite Chuck was. "I quickly reminded Rhonda of her own soldier!!"

We helped clean up and the soldiers settled at game tables. Before I knew it Rhonda was sitting with the girls all surrounding Blue Eyes while playing cards. I strolled by to give Rhonda my evil eye when blue eyes asked, "Hey do you want to learn how to play pinochle?"

"No. My daddy already taught me." I snobbishly replied.

"Awe, come on," he begged.

I put my nose in the air and walked straight through the double doors to the stage and dance hall. I checked to see if George's band, Round House, was posted yet and it was.

I sat and played Scrabble with Jim and could not believe how Rhonda was giggling and flirting with Blue Eyes. I won Scrabble and Jim had to get back to the base. I followed him out to see if George was there, because I had also promised Rhonda a ride home and I needed to get her away from Blue Eyes. I kept checking every ten minutes and George still hadn't shown.

Rhonda came over and asked, "Where is George? I have to get home."

Then Blue Eyes approached, "I don't mind giving you a ride home."

Rhonda hastily said, "Sure, Chuck that is so sweet of you."

We approached a 1967 Blue Rambler Rebel. Rhonda opened the front passenger door and I abruptly pushed her aside to sit next to Chuck so she would not sit next to him

"Sorry Rhonda, but I know you have to get home so we can drop you off first."

Rhonda rolled her eyes at me with disgust. Chuck made small talk about his father being stationed in Japan and was in the Air Force. I was so happy when he dropped off Rhonda that I slid right over to the window. Chuck did seem nice but I had to watch out for those soldiers in Vietnam and make sure their girls waited for them back in the States. He seemed a bit cocky and conceited, though. But nice, because he really had to go out of the way to take us both home.

"Thanks Chuck, I appreciate the ride."

"Awe, aren't you going to invite me in?"

"My mom said I can't bring anyone home for six months because I walked off the alter . . . . it's a long story . . ." I hesitated then gave in, "Okay you can come in but I don't think she will be very happy about it."

We entered the front door of our Georgia rancher and the lights were out in the front room but we heard the television in the back room.

"Mom, I'm home!" I called out. "George never showed to pick me up. So, Chuck gave me a ride home, but don't worry he is leaving now."

Mom came out of the family room and turned on the lights. She looked Chuck up and down and said, "Well hello there. You look like you could be one of my kids with that wavy hair and those big blue eyes! Come in and meet Marion's dad."

"Mom he is not staying he just gave me a ride."

"Nice to meet you, Sir," he said as he properly reached down his hand and shook Dad's hand.

I could have died. Dad had a roll of toilet paper at his side and had his head tilted due to a bloody nose.

Mom came running out of the kitchen with a plate of chocolate cake. "Here Chuck have some cake and visit awhile."

"Thank you so much." He became comfortable too fast and was chatting away about how his Dad was in the Air Force too and they also went to Japan. Then of course they shared their experiences in Japan.

Finally, Chuck said he needed to go.

I walked him to the porch and said goodnight.

"When will you be at the USO again?" He asked.

"I will be there with my friends Tuesday night. I have a really cool friend Barbara I want to introduce you to."

"Mom interrupted and said, "Now you come by any time you get lonesome."

Chuck waved as he climbed into his car.

I rushed to my mom, "Mom what happened to your 'no guy home for six month' rule? You act like he is my boyfriend, he is not my type. He might be nice but he is also conceited and cocky."

"Marion did you see those eyes? I just loved him!"

I rolled my eyes as I announced, "I am going to bed."

It was Tuesday and I could not wait to convince Barbara to date Chuck. We met in the restroom after DECCA class and she was excited. Barbara was a tall red head and quite attractive now that she had a nose job last summer. "Barbara, Chuck is about six feet tall, too tall for me! He is nice but not my type. Would you believe Rhonda, who didn't even want to go to the USO, fell for him? I was not about to let that happen!"

"I already heard about that from Rhonda. I guess she felt guilty and wrote her boyfriend a letter and told him all about it."

"I don't know if that was cool. Well, I plan on being there at six."

"Great, I invited Renee to come to. I am a little nervous."

I arrived a little early, Blue Eyes was already there. He was so happy to see me and came up to me as soon as I walked in the door, like he was waiting for me.

"Hi Chuck. Barbara will be here soon she is excited to meet you."

"Okay. How are your parents I sure liked them a lot."

"Good, Mom adored you. I reminded her though, no boyfriends for me."

He chuckled and said, "What's not to like about me?'

"You are so conceited!"

"Hey there is a band Friday night are you coming?"

"Yup, that is my brother's band playing. I kinda have to be his groupie!"

"Is that the brother that didn't pick you up?"

"That's him. He is a groovy drummer though!" "Well I will definitely be here then. I have to thank him for getting to know you better since you wouldn't play cards with me. I was happy to be your chauffer."

"Ha ha"

Our conversation was interrupted by Barbara and Renee.

"Chuck these are my friends Barbara and Renee."

I went to serve food and looked back to see them laughing. I was pleased that they seemed to get along so well. I must admit, I did enjoy Blue Eyes occasionally glancing over and smiling at me. It was like we were sharing an intimate plot. The girls left rather early and Chuck helped me clean up.

"Marion, the girls said they will be at the dance too."

"Good, then you can ask Barb out."

"Well I might need to talk to you about all this; can I have your phone number?"

"I guess so since we are friends."

"Let me get some pen and paper."

He returned to write down my phone number and walk me out.

"I will call you tomorrow."

I forgot to tell Chuck that I had a friendly date with Jim. When he called Mom answered the phone and told him I was out. I could not believe she invited him over to wait stating that I would not be out late. I came home shortly after a nice dinner with Jim where we shared all the USO gossip. I was shocked to see Chuck there and acting like he belonged there when I opened the door.

He had shared the whole story about me fixing him up with Barb. Before you knew we were all talking and laughing. I have to admit he had become quite comfortable and easy to talk to.

As I said goodnight I told him I would see him at the dance.

Chuck called Thursday night and asked me what he should wear to the dance.

"Jeans would be just fine."

"Okay I will go buy a pair."

"You don't have jeans?"

"No, my parents never allowed us to wear blue jeans."

"Wow they must have been strict!"

"Yah I was raised strict Southern Baptist."

"How old are you?"

"I will be 19 in April."

"Wow we are only 9 months apart!"

"Well I will see you tomorrow and I will introduce you to George," I continued.

"Good night."

I was so excited to go to the dance. I love to dance. I went to a little dress shop and bought a new dress. It was so perfect. It was a mini dress right in style with five gold chains draped on it. I had black stockings and platform heels to wear with it. I just wanted to dance the night away. I thought it would be fun with so many friends there as well as George and his band. I drove home to get ready and give Mom back her car.

Chuck called, "I can give you a ride home."

"Great I hate waiting for the band to pack up. Now, tonight you have to ask Barb out right?"

"Sure I will if you will come too."

"Now that wouldn't be a date." I thought about it, "Groovy I will see you there, bye."

The parking lot was already full when Mom dropped me off. I could see the band unloading all equipment.

"Marion have a great time and say hi to Chuck."

"Mom he is asking Barb out tonight, he is just my friend."

"Well what is wrong with him for you?'

I lifted my arms in the air and drew an invisible square. "He is a little too square for me and a little too conceited!"

"I don't think he is conceited just confident!"

"Besides he wears wing toed shoes, I even had to tell him to buy jeans for the dance!"

"Got to go Mom, see ya!"

I entered the crowded dance hall that rang with laughter and Chuck approached me first, "Wow you look so cool! I love that dress!"

"Thank-you Sir and you look pretty cool in those jeans." It was kind of cute the way he turned away when I complimented him. Then, without looking into my eyes he asked, "Are you going to save a dance for me?"

"Yes, I save a dance for everyone I am a USO girl!" The band started to play as Barb and Renee approached. We all found a table and sat together. Before I could sit down Jim approached me and asked me to dance. The band was playing *Black Magic Woman*, one of my favorites. I danced the night away the whole time thinking of how much I loved the purple dress. I saw Chuck dancing with both Barbara and Renee together. He caught my glance and smiled. The band slowed down the music and started playing *Summertime* and Chuck, once again not looking in my eyes, asked, "Can I have this dance?"

I smiled and awkwardly moved close to him. He took my hand to hold up in the air I could feel it quiver a little. I realized he was so much taller than me and I was grateful for my plat form shoes.

"The band is so good. Your brother is a fantastic drummer. Will you introduce me to him before we leave?"

"Sure, if you have a date with Barb!" I insisted.

"I do."

"Oh cool, where are you taking her and when?"

"We are going bowling, want to go?"

"No I am not going on your date!"

"Okay you will be missing a good time"

We both giggled and went back to the table. At the end of the evening I took Chuck over to meet George and the band. I could tell he was impressed to meet them. I told George that Chuck was taking me home.

We pulled in front of my house.

"Now you have a great time on your date and call me when you get back to the barracks!"

"Okay or maybe I will just stop by."

"Cool. Goodnight." I got out of the car and waved as he drove off. I was too tired to talk anymore but realized how easy he was to talk to. We had become good friends.

I had to work at the hospital all day Saturday. I was so happy to be transferred to the emergency room. The time went by so much faster and it is exciting. If I became a nurse I would definitely wanted to be an ER nurse. After work, I went by my friend Karen's house to share all my drama with finding Chuck a date, she was much taller than I with long, straight, blonde hair and green eyes. Straight hair was in style. I was a bit jealous. Even rolling my hair in orange juice cans wouldn't take the curl out of my hair. She was a great listener. We both had Catholic families with six kids. Since I did not go to Warner Robins High anymore due to rezoning of the school district, we didn't have a lot of friends in common.

Her brother's friend "Richard" was about to go into the Navy and she was devastated, She was determined that he would fall in love with her.

"Marion it sounds like you really like Chuck. Why are you fixing him up?"

"Like my mom says, he is so nice! We are just friends."

"Well Richard thinks we are just friends, but when he comes home I am going to marry him."

"Well if I marry Blue Eyes you will be the first to know!" I went home to play records and wait for Chuck to call. I even baked a cake because I was certain he would come by. I kept looking out the window and no car lights. Every time the phone rang I jumped to get it.

Mom asked, "And why aren't you out with him? It looks like you more than just like him to me!"

"Mom, he's really not my type." I drew a square in the air to remind her. "I don't like how he dresses and he is almost too nice. But I do love talking to him and yes he does have beautiful eyes!"

"Okay, if he asks I will go out on a date with him! That is if he didn't fall in love with Barb tonight because he is not here and didn't call. The phone rang and I ran to get it. Mom waved goodnight with a pleasant smile on her face as I said "Hello Woods Residence."

"Hi Marion, it was too late to come by, I just got back to the barracks." My cheeks flushed and my heart raced with excitement that he had called.

Lying, I responded, "I hope you had a good time on your date with Barb."

"It was fun, but it would have been more fun if you came."

"I was not about to share your date."

"Why not? Barb brought Renee."

"Oh man, they really are glued at the hip!"

"We had a lot of laughs though. I went on a date now can I take you out? Just us?"

"I guess so. Where are we going?" I asked, trying to hide my enthusiasm.

"There is a carnival outside of the base and I get paid Friday. I can win you a teddy bear."

"That does sound like fun!"

"I can't wait. It's a date see you Saturday at 6:00. During the day I have to coach little league with my Sergeant."

"Cool, you coach baseball. You must like kids."

"Love them. I want 11 so I can have my own football team!"

"Wow, impressive good luck finding a woman to have 11 kids!"

"You mean you don't want eleven kids?"

"I really want a big family but maybe not quite that many".

We both burst into laughter!

"Marion Woods I like you!"

"Chuck, what's your last name?"

"Barnes."

"Well Chuck Barnes, I like you too!"

"I better get off here; I don't want your parents to get mad. See ya Saturday!"

"Bye." I had a hard time falling asleep that night. I realized I was falling for blue eyes.

I knew I had to talk to Karen. I went over mid week. Her family invited me for spaghetti. I think it was southern style but I loved the way the peppers and onions smelled simmering in their kitchen. I couldn't wait for dinner to end so Karen and I could go for a walk and talk in private.

As soon as we got on the front porch I started running at the mouth.

"Karen, he asked me out and I said yes!"

"What, I thought you were fixing him up?"

"I did, but she took a friend and I was actually excited that it wasn't romantic."

"Man, I knew it!"

"Karen he told me he wanted eleven kids. What if I can't have kids? What will he be like knowing I don't have a bellybutton? I am freaking out!"

"Marion he isn't falling for your bellybutton, it is your personality!"

"Karen there were several reasons I walked off the alter away from Ralph. I don't want to make that mistake again. Did you know he was afraid I wouldn't be able to have sex because of my surgeries?" I continued on, "Karen after we broke up I had sex to prove him wrong and to prove to myself that I was capable. I hope God forgives me. Chuck will hate me for not being a virgin!"

"Oh my God, Marion, I can't believe you had sex with that creep!" You need to go to confession Saturday. God will forgive you, that was special circumstances. Anyone that falls in love with you will forgive you. Chuck sounds so nice I know he will understand."

"Guess what?!" She asked excitedly. "Richard is writing me back from the Navy!"

"Karen that is so cool!"

"You know I am going to marry him!"

We both laughed. Karen reminded me she had homework and we called it a night. I loved her confidence in me! I was scared of a relationship but I knew I would try again. I couldn't wait until Saturday.

Saturday finally arrived. I just had to get through working at the hospital and then date time. When I arrived home my younger sisters, Patty and Ruthie, ran to greet me.

"Marion, Chuck was at the BX with us today."

Patty hurriedly told Ruthie, "Shhh it's a secret." Patty was six years younger than I. She was an adorable stylish twelve-year old with long, wavy, sandy blonde hair. She was serious about her school work and seemed to admire me; Ruthie had long, darker, wavy hair with pink cheeks and bright blue eyes. She was always full of laughter. Most girls were annoyed by their younger sisters, but I adored mine. Mom always bought Ruthie blue clothes and Patty pink clothes. Sometime I thought of them as dolls. Today I was annoyed because they would not confide in me why Mom and Chuck were together. I gave up and went in my room to prepare for my date. It was a few minutes before six when Chuck rang the door bell. No one would answer. I heard the girls and Mom calling my name to answer the door. Annoyed I went to the door and swung it open. There stood Chuck with this proud grin on his face as he said, "Hi!"

My mouth fell wide open. There he was dressed in a white pair of bell bottoms with a beach boy striped shirt and he was wearing the coolest sandals.

Mom blurted out, "He doesn't look too square now does he?"

Patty chimed in, "Mom picked out some cool clothes!"

Ruthie squealed, "She sure did!" Before I could reply Mom shooed us out the door telling us to have fun.

"Chuck you do look cool," I admitted.

"Thanks it took a lot of help from your Mom. I love your family!"

"Me too," I agreed. We arrived at the carnival grounds. It was a little dusty, I thought, for those white bell bottom pants but he sure looked cool in them. Chuck reached down and held my hand. I got butterflies in my stomach. It was just like when Alan had held my hand. From that point on, every time I heard the song, *Close to You* by the Carpenters, I thought of Chuck, and that song seemed to play a lot!

"Well I told you I was going to win you a teddy bear. There are games over there."

To no avail he couldn't win a thing. He was spending far too much money trying even after I reassured him that I did not need a prize. Finally, he won me a soft brown eyed teddy bear with a red ribbon around its neck. We enjoyed the evening and he took me home late.

We parked in front of my parent's house and he asked if he could kiss me goodnight. He put his gentle hands around me to slide me close to him. His kiss was gentle upon my lips and I did not want to stop kissing but I had to pull away.

"I need to get in but call me and thanks for my bear I love him!"
"Think of me when you sleep with him tonight!"
"I think I will, he will be my Chuckie poo!"
"No I want to be your Chuckie poo!"
"Okay good night Chuckie poo!"

Mom was so excited about us dating that she immediately invited him to dinner. It was obvious that she wanted him to be part of the family. I baked stuffed chickens and Chuck came over and made a cherry pie. I could have died when we had no napkins and Mom put a roll of toilet paper on the table. Chuck burst into laughter but seemed to enjoy every moment. It was time for dessert and he dished out his cherry pie. It was horrible!

He forgot the sugar. "Mom said, oh Chuck I love it! I don't like that much sugar in my pie." Everyone else avoided the pie as we laughed at her comment. It was another fun day and another wonderful goodnight kiss. We talked every night; we were together as much as possible.

It was the Friday before Good Friday when it hit me. I never had my monthly period.

I began to panic. Even going to confession couldn't fix this. I called Karen to come over after school. Her Mom dropped her off and I swept her away into my bedroom.

"Karen I think I might be pregnant. I am so sad because I am falling in love with Chuck! How will I ever tell him or even worse Mom and Dad?"

"Oh my God is it that creep's?"

"It couldn't be anyone else. Chuck will break up with me and Mom and Dad will be so disappointed."

"Marion you have no choice but to tell them. At least tell your parents now and maybe later, Chuck. You have to think of the baby."

"I know. I would love a baby but I would rather it not be Ralph's!"

"Promise me you will tell them!"

"I will tell my mom tomorrow but what if they want Ralph to marry me?"

"I did not think about that. Let's just see what happens." It was time for her to leave so I took Mom's car and drove Karen home, I told her as I dropped her off, "I am so glad we are friends."

"Me too! Call me and let me know what happens."

It was a pretty day and I did not want to ruin it with my drama. Dad was fixing his famous breakfast. I love the smell of the bacon frying, After breakfast I helped clean up and Dad went out to work on his new project, building designer dog houses. Patty and Ruthie went out to play with their friend Connie. George went into the garage to set up his band equipment with his buddy Bruce and Kenny and Johnny had ball practice. There was no excuse I had Mom in the backroom all alone.

"Mom, can I talk to you about something really serious?"

"Marion what's wrong?"

"Mom I did something so bad, I am so sorry, I know it is a sin, I had sex with Ralph." I started to cry.

"Oh my God! Did he hurt you?"

"No he didn't hurt me, it was the night I walked off the alter . . . Mom I do not love him!"

"I know you don't."

"Mom I missed my period, I am so afraid that I am pregnant.

"Marion you have always been irregular and we will deal with all of this. You have been under so much stress lately with the wedding mess, getting ready for graduation and working. I will call the base and schedule you an appointment for after Easter. Marion it will all work out!" Then she wrapped me in her arms and I knew she forgave me and it would be okay.

The phone rang. Mom answered and said, "It's Chuck for you." Then she covered the phone piece and asked in a whisper, "Does he know?" I shook my head and whispered back "No." I wiped the tears from my eyes and cheerfully as possible said "Hi Chuck."

"Hi Marion. I am so excited I have tickets for the Kenny Rogers and the First Edition concert Friday, do you want to go?"

"Cool that sounds like fun. I would love to go. It's Good Friday but I can go to mass early.

"I will pick you up at six."

"Okay that is great. Bye."

Concerned Mom said, "There is no need to tell him until you know for certain."

The following evening I decided against Mom's advice that I did need to talk to Chuck. We met at Shoney's drive-in. I climbed in his car as he was ordering our strawberry pie and onion rings to split.

"Hi, you sounded so serious when you called. Is everything okay?"

"No. I hate telling you this. Well, you know I walked off the alter before marring Ralph because he was such a jerk."

"And I am glad you did!"

Bursting out in tears I muttered, "I think I may be pregnant."

"Oh, it's okay, don't cry." He put his arms around me to comfort me.

"I can't believe I had sex with him."

"I don't care, I love you and I want to marry you whether you're pregnant or not!"

"Marry me, but that is not all that is wrong with me, I don't even have a bellybutton!"

"You don't need a bellybutton to get married!"

"I love you too!"

"Okay no one has to know the baby belongs to Ralph, I will love it as my own."

"I go to the doctors next week after Easter and I will find out."

"So let's have fun at the concert and not worry. We will have a great Easter."

He kissed me tenderly and had convinced me all was going to be okay. We enjoyed a piece of pie together. I kissed him goodnight and told him I was so excited about the concert. He did not need anymore worry or tears from me.

Friday was finally here. I had no school or work. My friend Jim called and asked if I was going to the USO. I had been so busy with Chuck and my own drama that I had neglected my friendship with Jim. I promised I would be over at lunch time. I pulled up right at noon and Jim met me at the car.

"Marion it is a beautiful day to sit outside, let's walk to the park."

"It is nice out and I would love to walk to the park." We walked around to the park and we rested on a park bench.

"Well Marion, what or who has been keeping you so busy?"

"You know I have school and my work at the hospital. Yes, and okay I have been dating Chuck a lot!"

"Well he is really a nice guy and if he hasn't asked you to marry you yet I want to."

"You want to marry me?!"

"Yes I do."

"You know I am not ready to marry anyone after all that mess with Ralph."

"Well I am not Ralph and I do not want Chuck to steal you away!"

"You are so sweet! I just have so much going on in my life right now. You are such a good friend and I am so honored."

"I guess that is a *no* for now. I won't give up." We both laughed and walked back into the USO, we visited with everyone and then I had to leave for mass and then the concert.

During church, I knew I should be thanking God for sending his son Jesus to save us but I kept praying for peace and forgiveness. I was not sure what I should do. When I left mass I hurried home to get ready to go to the concert before Chuck arrived.

I started to feel cramping in my abdomen. I went to the bathroom and discovered blood. I cried tears of joy and sadness. I knew God answered my prayers but the thought of a baby did warm my heart. All I ever wanted was a family. I ran and told Mom. I could tell she shared my same emotions. I loved Mom and Dad for the support they had given me.

"Mom, thanks for all your help."

"Marion you better take some aspirin if you are going to the concert."

"Okay I will."

"Mom I saw Jim at the USO today. He wanted to know why I was always so busy."

"What did you tell him?'

"I told him school and work and that I was dating Chuck."

"Good, we love Chuck."

"Mom, he said he wanted me to marry him if Chuck hadn't asked me already."

"Wow!"

"I told him I was not ready yet because I need to graduate and I had so much going on in my life."

"That was a good answer." Our conversation was interrupted by the doorbell.

"Well hi there Chuck!" Mom greeted him so cheerfully. I ran to my room to freshen up my make-up and get a jacket.

Mom yelled, "Have a good time," as we got into the car.

We climbed to the top of the bleachers to have a good view. The music was awesome. I could hardly wait for it to end though to tell Chuck the news.

He was singing along to all the songs. They sounded a bit country to me. I was familiar with *Ruby Don't Take Your Love To Town* "and *"Ruben James."* I felt cool being at my first concert. The music ended and Chuck said, "Let's sit here until the traffic clears out."

The crowd slowly moved toward their cars and it was quiet enough to start a conversation.

"Chuck I have some news, I started my period. You do not have to marry me now."

"Marion I didn't want to marry you just because you thought you were pregnant. I want to marry you because I love you! I am going to ask your Dad on Easter Sunday if I can ask you to marry me," he paused, "If you will have me."

"Yes Chuck I will marry you!" We kissed fervently in the humid air.

"Marion," he said, pulling back. "Let's get you home or your Dad will say no!" On the drive home, my heart must have raced a mile a minute.

"This has been some day. Would you believe Jim said he wanted to marry me if you didn't?" I smiled at him reassuringly, "I told him I was not ready. But, he is going to be shocked when I tell him I am marring you!"

"He better not try to steal my girlfriend. I like him though he has good taste like I do in women."

"I love *you* Chuck!"

"We can tell him together okay?"

"Okay kiss me goodnight. I'll see you on Easter!"

Saturday Mom and I went shopping. I found the cutest Easter dress. It was white on top with puffed sleeves, umpire waist with a light blue bottom. It was short but so cute. I knew chuck would love it. Mom was picking up candy for all of our baskets. I was so tempted to tell her what Chuck was going to ask Dad tomorrow but I didn't want to ruin the surprise. I think she will be so pleased because she adores him. The day went by so fast.

I got up Easter morning and heard all the kid's excited voices yelling, "Marion get up the Easter bunny came!" Here I was 18 years old and I was still excited to see if I had a basket. I put on my robe and went into the living room. Not only did I have a basket but there was one for Chuck, too! I started laughing as I opened it. Inside was a bubble pipe, chocolate bunny, jelly beans and new kite.

"Mom, I am eighteen!"

"You are still my little girl and I love your Chuckie Poo!"

"I think he will love his basket, too!"

"He will be here soon. We are going to Debbie's church in Bonaire at eleven."

"I am going to go get dressed!" When I came out Chuck was already there and Mom had just given him his Easter basket. Chuck laughed but his eyes were teary, "I haven't had one of these since I was about eight. Thank you." We left to go to church. Chuck had parked down the street and we had to walk a little. I looked back and saw Mom waving bye at us.

"After lunch I am going to ask your Dad. Do you still want to marry me?"

"More than ever." He squeezed my hand and off to church we went.

It was a beautiful day. All the kids were outside and we heard Mom and Dad in the backroom talking. Chuck took my hand and led me back to Mom and Dad.

"Sergeant Woods, may I have your daughter's hand in marriage?"

"Yes, you may if she will have you!" He replied tearfully and joyfully.

Chuck fell to his knees and in front of me and asked, "Marion will you marry me?"

"Yes!"

Chuck jumped up and lifted me in the air to hug him. Unlike with Ralph I looked over at Mom and saw tears of joy in her eyes. Dad went to his bar and brought out a bottle of champagne. He popped the cork and when it hit the ceiling he started to cry.

"Chuck, welcome to the family you can now call me Dad or Woodsie no more Sergeant Woods." It was a glorious Easter Day!

I was on my way to school when Mom reminded me, "Don't forget your doctor appointment is tomorrow at two. This is so important especially now that you will be getting married. Every girl needs a pre-marital checkup."

"Okay but I hate going to the doctors!"

I was so excited to tell all my friends that Chuck had proposed. Some seemed excited and others thought it was too soon. Barbara asked, "Why were you trying to fix him up with me?"

"I just did not think I was ready for a relationship."

"Well he is a great guy! You are a very lucky girl! I would have tried harder, but I have college ahead of me."

"You are so smart you need to go to college. We want to get married and have lots of kids!"

"I hope I am invited to the wedding!"

"You know you are."

The warm Georgia sun was starting to set when I realized I had to call Debbie and ask her to be my matron of honor since I was hers. I spent so much time gloating and daydreaming but now it was time to act and get things organized and ready.

"Hi Debbie!" I said cheerfully and before she could respond, I continued, "Guess what? Chuck proposed! I am so happy! Will you be my Matron of Honor?"

Debbie replied with her soft southern accent, "Of course I will. He is so nice!"

"This time I want to do it my way. I want a reception at the house and flowers from the yard. My friend Renate has a beautiful white empire dress she said I could borrow. There is no way Mom and Dad should have to go into debt. I just want it simple!"

"That does sound more like you instead of that other gown and the ballroom at the club on base. "So when is the date?"

"We will figure all that out this weekend. Now I just have to get through tomorrow. Mom has made me an appointment for a pre-marital check up."

"Yuck, good luck! Call me with the details. We will get together soon."

"Okay we'll do!"

Chapter 6

I woke up dreading my appointment but ready to get it over with. Mom picked me up at school and drove straight to the clinic. I guess because of all my surgeries I feared hospitals. The scent of alcohol was present and the wall was all a dull green. The tile floors were over waxed giving such a sterile appearance. Mom checked out my records and we walked to the clinic.

"Marion hold the records while you're waiting to be called. I have to use the restroom." I randomly glanced through them out of curiosity and to kill time. The words on the page jumped right out to me "undetermined sex." Oh my God what does that mean? It means I am a freak! Frantically, I read further: Biopsy revealed patient as female. So did that mean I looked like a male? My mind raced with awful doubts and insecurities. Mom had returned but I was too uncomfortable and shocked to discuss my revelation.

The nurse called, "Marion Woods."

"Mom whispered, "I will wait out here." The nurse escorted me to the examining room and gave me directions, "Please remove your clothing and climb on the table placing your feet in the stirrups."

The room was cold and I was shivering; I was relieved to see the doctor come in shortly after. As performed the exam, he kept muttering what an amazing job Boston Children's had done. After what seemed like an eternity, the exam was completed. The doctor told me to dress and come into his office. Then he said he was going to ask Mom to join us.

Mom was already sitting in front of the desk and I sat beside her. He addressed me as Miss Woods. I was starting to feel grown up.

"Miss Woods I hear you are about to be married soon."

I replied, "Yes, hopefully in June."

"Do you plan on having children?"

"Well yes. My fiancé jokes about having his own football team."

In a concerning voice, he proceeded, "You have had a tremendous amount of experimental but successful surgery. I am assuming with this much surgery you could have built up a serious amount of scar tissue that would prevent a pregnancy. If you do become pregnant you may have trouble carrying full term because your hips are wired together. Once again," he paused, "I have no other cases to compare this to so we just don't know for sure. However you need to be aware of the possible complications. I wish you the best of luck in your marriage."

Mom and I walked back to the car. I did not want to talk at all. I felt as if my life was crumbling down around me. To think I once thought that not having a bellybutton was the worst thing in the world, but the possibility of no children devastated me. Mom broke the silence as we shut the car door. "Marion you need to tell Chuck everything the doctor told you today."

"I know I do but, maybe I shouldn't marry him. He wants a large family."

"Marion if he is the right guy for you it will all work out."

"I am going out with him tomorrow night and I will tell him then." All the next day I was in a daze. I panicked about talking to Chuck. I contemplated breaking up. Inevitably, I did have to face the music and talk with him. He promptly showed up at 5:30. I answered the doorbell and smiled at his enthusiasm to treat me to Shoney's Big Boy, a drive-in restaurant where the girls delivered the food on roller skates. He almost made me forget about my news. Quickly I ushered him to the car to prevent him and Mom from getting into a deep conversation. I wanted to handle this all by myself. Chuck ordered for us both and then questioned, "Well how did your appointment go?"

I lost control and burst into tears, as I babbled my story, "Chuck, I cannot marry you. The doctor said I may not be able to have children and you want a big family. You would be stuck with a wife with no bellybutton and no kids. You do not deserve that. I love you too much to marry you!"

He pulled a handkerchief out from his pocket and gently dried my eyes and told me to stop crying.

"I love you so much even if you do not have a bellybutton. We can always adopt kids. All I know is that I want to be your husband. We are going to get married no matter what." Our food arrived by the waitress on roller skates. He paid her and took our burgers off the tray, "This is a lot of food. Don't make me eat it alone. Just say you will be my wife and let's eat."

"Are you sure?"

"Yes I am surer of marrying you than anything in my life!"

"Yes I will be your wife. Let's eat!" Mom anxiously waited up to hear how Chuck had accepted the news. I told her he still wanted us to wed. She acknowledged with a simple, "I knew it! Now off to bed we have a graduation and wedding to plan for!"

The weekend came and all the plans were made. I graduated high school on June 4, 1971. I married Chuck on June 5, 1971. It was the only date we could book the church. With all the excitement and emotions, it felt like we were on a roller coaster ride. We made lists for invitations and graduation announcements. Mom, who never sewed, decided she would make the bridesmaid gowns for my sisters. I could not imagine them not being in my wedding because of the cost of dresses. I just adored them so much. The wedding colors were purple and pink.

My cap and gown for graduation was white. Chuck loved the excitement and was easy going with all the plans. He loved that we were getting married by a Protestant minister instead of a priest. Our plans were done and Chuck promised that the next weekend we would spend time alone.

The following weekend was not a military pay day so Chuck was short on cash so we decided to go on a picnic. All I could find in the refrigerator was bologna and I made grape Kool-Aid. The basket was packed with bologna sandwiches, chips and marshmallows for dessert. My mind kept drifting back to the doctor's appointment. I could not get the word undetermined sex out of my mind. I was becoming obsessed with having a baby to prove I was a woman and not a freak. I did know that Chuck really loved me no matter what but I still was not sure about this being the right thing to do.

Chuck arrived at the house and came in with a big smile.

He whispered in my ear, "I brought a blanket for our picnic."

I smiled, "Well lunch is all packed let's go!" We drove outside of town. We wanted a quiet special place.

Chuck announced "I found it look!"

Sitting before us was a meadow surrounded by a wooded area with large weeping willow trees. The sun made it glow like a majestic place.

"Chuck it looks like a picture out of the Bambi book."

"It does! Look over there!" I looked where he pointed and saw a dear scampering through the meadow. We walked until we found a perfect place to lay our blanket.

I unpacked our lunch. Chuck relished his sandwiches.

"How did you know I love bologna?"

"Well wait to you see what is for dessert!"

"Uh marshmallows, that is not my favorite unless they are in hot chocolate!"

I packed up our leftovers as he lay down on the blanket. "Chuck let's go for a walk. It is so peaceful and beautiful here."

"Later, come lay down by my side." I went and laid my head on his shoulder. He passionately kissed me. I loved kissing him back. He reached down and pulled up my shirt. Panicked, I pulled my shirt back down. I fearfully whispered, "Chuck my scars and remember: no bellybutton."

"Marion, it's okay. I love all of you." Then he proceeds to lift my blouse and caress and kiss all my scars so tenderly. That was the moment I knew I wanted to marry this wonderful man. I was filled with love and joy. I had similar feelings for Alan. That was something I never had expected to experience again. I knew I was glowing brighter than the sun. The butterflies around us must have flown right into my stomach!

Chuck stood up and helped me up. "Now let's go for a walk. Maybe I can find a fishing hole around here.

We walked less than a half of mile when we discovered the town dump. We both burst into laughter. Our magical, majestic place was by the dump.

The sun was starting to set so it was time to go home. I was leaving that day feeling like a real woman. Soon, I would be graduating but even that could not be as special as that day.

Graduation day was here. Our whole family was attending, Dad made sure to bring his sunglasses to hide any tears. All my siblings shared my enthusiasm. The ceremony was held outdoors at the high school stadium. Chuck planned on meeting us there. When I got into line for the ceremony I did not see him. I knew there was time because my last name was "W."

So many people had gathered that I could not recognize anyone. Finally my name was called. Having a big family made me sound popular with all the yelling. I stepped down the platform after receiving my diploma and out of nowhere Chuck came forth and picked me up to carry me to my family.

It was a beautiful sunny day, but a little too hot. The high was supposed to reach 105 degrees. I could already hear Mom working in the kitchen. It smelled wonderful. She cooked all the food for the reception at the house. I couldn't contain all my excitement. Chuck had snuck back in the house after the graduation party even though everyone said it would be bad luck to see the bride before the wedding day. Mom ran him off about 1:00 am. He stayed at the little city hall apartment that we rented a week earlier. My younger brother Johnny came bursting into the house. He rode his bike over and took pictures of Chuck.

Johnny entered my room, "Marion, he must love you because he is doing handstands in front of your house!" Then he snickered, "Me, George and Kenny are in charge of decorating the car. Don't think Chuck'll like that." He broke into a devilish laugh. It was quite contagious.

"Well I am glad he is happy. I know he keeps expecting his parents to show but they are stationed in Japan." I peeked out the front window then told Johnny, "Get out of my room now. I have a lot to do. Scram!" I cleaned my room and laid out my wedding dress. I took a long hot bath and then went to get my hair done. When I arrived back home, my matron of honor was already there. They came straight to the room to help me dress. Mom was dressing Patty and Ruthie in the lovely lavender dotted Swiss gowns she had made. Debbie wore my pink prom dress. I felt gorgeous in my white gown with an opal beaded umpire waist. I put on my vale and couldn't wait to show Mom. There she stood with rollers in her hair and shorts on. She looked up at me and began to cry; she lifted my vale and kissed me telling me how beautiful I looked. It was another magic moment. We took pictures and she told me to go to the church with Dad. She had to get ready and would follow.

"Marion I am almost out of gas and we need to find a gas station," Dad said apologetically. I was melting in my gown. Just then the truck started to sputter thank God we were right in front of a gas station.

We pulled up to the church and waited for Mom. She was on time and we entered the church. I am sure everyone was recalling the last time when I never made it down the isle. That was not going to happen this time! *Here Comes The Bride* started to play and I walked down the isle. This time I allowed Dad to give me away. Chuck took my hand into his quivering hand. We said our vows and were pronounced *Man and Wife*.

The reception was so much fun. The food amazed everyone, it was so good. We could not wait to go to our little house. Dad threw grass seed instead of rice. We did not have enough money for a honeymoon but we didn't care.

Chapter 7

Our first little house was decorated cute with little knickknacks from my room and a few wedding gifts. Even though it was nice to have the apartment furnished, we couldn't use the bed because it was moldy, so we slept on the coach. In our minds, it was perfect. I did freak out when slugs came out in the middle of the night. As the weeks went by we received wedding checks. Chuck decided we could take a honeymoon at his Aunt's house in Florida with the money. I felt strange leaving the state without Mom and Dad, but we were so excited.

Chuck's Aunt welcomed us with open arms. Her home was close to Fort Walton Beach. It was decorated so beautifully and quite immaculate. Best of all there was a pool out back. Our room was large and very comfortable. We could not wait until the next day to go to the beach. We held hands and walked along the whitest sand I had ever seen. In the midst of the beauty, some dead fish washed ashore and I vomited right on the beach.

"Marion are you okay?"

"It is just that horrible smell," I complained.

"Awe it's not that bad! How am I going to take you fishing?"

"Chuck I am so hungry. I really want some pizza!"

"You just threw up are you sure? It is only 11:00am in the morning," he pointed out.

"Well maybe that is why the smell got to me. But, I need pizza," I insisted.

"Let's walk down the beach farther—there are some restaurants." We walked farther down and all we could find open was a hamburger place. We took our food and ate on the beach. We stayed out there until the sun began to set. It was an astonishing day. We went back to shower and we were so burnt. We couldn't even touch each other in bed. The weekend getaway ended much too quickly.

On the ride home we kept seeing fruit stands. I told Chuck I needed peaches to take home. But, before we arrived home I had eaten all the peaches. The next few weeks construction workers were tarring the road close to the house. Every time I got wind of the smell, I had to vomit. Chuck decided it was not a normal reaction.

"Marion aren't women suppose to have periods every month?"

"Yes but I am irregular, remember?"

"Well, I think you need to go talk to your Mom tonight." I called Mom and she invited us for dinner. When it quieted down I explained my vomiting.

"Mom do you think I might be pregnant?"

"Marion I believe you are homesick. Your life has changed so much. You have also been on a trip. Remember the doctors think it would be very difficult to get pregnant. It may never happen. You probably just want it so bad you believe you are pregnant."

We went home and discussed what Mom believed.

"Chuck I hate to throw up! There is no way I would make myself do that but maybe Mom is right."

"Marion there is a guy I work with. He just found out his wife is pregnant. She just took her urine to the hospital after being two months late and they call you in three days."

"Even though I'm irregular, I am three months late."

"I will call the clinic tomorrow to see where we go."

I tried not to get my hopes up but Mom was right I wanted a baby so badly. We took in a urine specimen to the clinic. The three day wait was treacherous. We decided not to tell Mom until the test results were in. We were to call in at noon on Friday. We did not have a phone but we could walk to the gas station to call. I hated to do it alone but I would. At 11:45 Chuck came charging in the door.

"I took the day off so we can celebrate our baby!"

"I may not be pregnant though."

"Then I will be here for you because I know how sad you will be." Together we drove to the phone booth. Chuck took the phone number and change into the booth. I followed anxiously and stood outside. I saw his arm reach up in the air and come down as if someone had just scored a home run. He came out of the booth and I stared at him anxiously.

"I am going to be a Dad and you are going to be a Mom!"

"I am pregnant?"

"Yes you are. Let's go tell your parents they are going to be grandparents!" As we drove down Watson Boulevard Chuck started yelling at the window, "We are having a baby!" to every car and person we passed. I was amazed at his reaction and loving every moment. All I could think was that I was a woman. Dad was not home yet and the kids were at school. Mom's reaction was cautious repeating, "Are you sure?" Chuck explained to her that the test was done on base and that we had an appointment for the doctors the following week.

I knew Mom was worried about her baby, me. I also knew God had answered all my prayers and everything was going to be perfect. We stayed until Dad got home and of course Chuck had to do the announcement.

"Dad, you are going to be a Grandpa." Dad, who was still in his Air Force uniform broke into tears and hugged Chuck who was still in his uniform. I looked at Mom who let down her guard and was also in tears. We went home not as newly weds but expectant parents.

The pregnancy was determined high risk. I watched my diet and ate healthy. I was determined to deliver this baby. Morning sickness seemed to never end. As I approached the last semester of my pregnancy the doctors were shocked. They informed us the clinic would not be prepared for such a complicated birth. They made plans to send us to a regional military hospital in Biloxi, Mississippi. Chuck was upset that they were sending me alone. He arranged to have orders to go with me. Mom and Dad were so excited they were driving down once we told them the day of the scheduled c-section. I meticulously packed a pink baby outfit and a blue one. Everyone was happy and excited but underneath I was scared.

The hospital was quite large and well equipped. Several different doctors ran tests for eleven long days. Chuck visited several times a day. I was quite mobile but I needed to stay in the vicinity of the hospital.

"Chuck I am going stir crazy. They still haven't told me the date of the c-section. Tomorrow is New Years Eve. I want to go dancing! I am fine!" A nurse over heard me whining and interrupted, "Airman Barnes, occasionally the doctors issue passes. Would you like to request one for New Years Eve?"

"Yes ma'am, I would love that! Marion, are you sure you're up to this?"

"That would be so cool!" The nurse left to file the request.

We were thrilled when the request was granted. There were some stipulations. We could not leave the base and had to return by midnight. If I had any discomfort I needed to return immediately.

"Man it is going to be great to get out of this room. We can go to the recreation center. Is there one on base?"

"I will plan a wonderful evening for us. Maybe we can have our baby on New Year's Day!" The following day couldn't come fast enough. The doctor visited earlier in the morning and told us the c-section was planned for January 4th. We then had two things to celebrate till midnight. First on the agenda was to call Mom and Dad so they could travel down. I put on a polyester purple maternity outfit and we went on our date.

Chuck took me to the club for a steak dinner. We conversed through the whole meal. Then, we danced the night away. I don't think the doctors would have approved.

Like Cinderella, I had to be home before the clock struck twelve. I was so tired and it was a long walk to the hospital.

"Marion I feel cheated; no labor, no getting you to the hospital in time. Everything is so planned out."

"You are right that isn't fair! That base police car would give us a ride if I was in labor!"

"Are you sure you don't feel any pain?" On that note, I started to bend over and rub my stomach and groan a little. The care did a complete u-turn and came to the rescue.

The young sergeant rolled down the window and in a panic asked, "Can I give you a ride to the hospital?"

"Yes sir that is exactly where we need to be. Thank you sir." Chuck assisted me into the car. "We are almost there. It is going to be all right."

Chuck thanked the sergeant once again and he drove away. Immediately we both burst into laughter.

"Now Chuck was that enough excitement for you?"

"It will do. It is certainly a story we will tell our child!" We giggled all the way back to my room. Chuck tucked me in and kissed me a tender New Years kiss.

January 4th arrived with a great visit from Mom and Dad before I was taken to surgery. I felt less frightened after seeing Mom's smile and Dad's teary eyes. I was given an epidural and had a bad reaction. As soon as they told me I had a healthy baby boy, they put me fast to sleep to recover. I had a migraine and an infection. I was on my back for three days and I was unable to see the baby. When I started to recover, they put me in a semi-private room. The nurse brought me the baby. I was so happy to see he had Chuck's beautiful blue eyes. They took him to the nursery and Chuck came in. He was only allowed to view him through a window. That made me so sad because I was not able to hold him for very long.

"Marion I love you so much. I was so scared. Can you believe we have a son? I want him to be Charles Richard Barnes Junior."

"Okay but I am going to call him Ricky! Charles is a little too stuffy!" Our world broadened with Ricky in it. I wondered if he would ever know what his birth meant to me. He validated me as a woman. I was placed in a new room with another young mother. She had her baby girl early all alone. Her husband was in Vietnam. We were thrilled to give her the little girl dress we brought to be prepared if we had a girl. I thought it brightened her spirit a little bit. This war had played havoc with so many lives. No sooner had I given her the dress her husband, dressed in full military uniform walked into the room. The joy on her face lit up our dull room. When she cried I cried. Goose bumps ran over my body. They allowed him to return early. I wished that moment could be shared with every civilian and not all the war negativity. We who lived this life knew the burdens our families and loved ones endured to protect our liberty.

Chapter 8

We loved being parents. Chuck would often get a little forlorn unable to share his joy with his parents. One weekend he called his grandmother in North Carolina. He was thrilled to hear his parents were returning from Japan. They wanted us to visit all of them in a couple of weeks. They informed us that there was to be a big family reunion picnic as well. Chuck was so excited but soon realized we did not have any funds to travel. I knew we had to find away. We put our brains together and realized the only thing we had of value was my record player coffee table that Mom and Dad had given me when I was a teen younger.

"Marion you can't sell that."

"Yes I can! I am going to go call Mom." I called her and her beautiful reply was, "A gift is a gift. It is yours to do what you wish. I know how you love hearing your records. Chuck does need to see his parents though." I was so thrilled to tell Chuck to sell my record player. A couple from work bought it and we had our travel funds.

We journeyed off to North Carolina. We went to his grandma's house. It was a large southern white farm house surrounded by beautiful trees. The house had a complete wrap around porch. I was so nervous that I think it made Ricky cranky. Chuck told me that his Mom liked ladies well groomed with short hair. I took offense until I understood he wanted them to love me like he did. There was a lot of gossip shared with us by his cousin that he married a Yankee and a Catholic at that. I had butterflies flipping in my stomach as we entered the front door. His little brother Dennis came and hugged him followed by his Dad. His mother and grandma followed with little side hugs. Chuck introduced me and Ricky.

"Charles, give me that baby. He sounds hungry." His mother had such a strong southern accent. I didn't expect that being in the military for over 25 years. I followed her into the big country kitchen. There was a large wooden bowl for making biscuits. You could tell a lot of southern food had been prepared there. His grandmother was quiet. Both women focused on Ricky stating he was much too thin. I was amazed to find out that his grandmother had twelve children Chuck enjoyed sharing his memories and showing off all the pictures. I was not used to everyone calling him Charles. I was happy to have the evening wind down so we could retire and relax. I was still so nervous. The next day would be more relaxing going to the park for his dad's family reunion.

I woke early to bathe and put on my wig that I used from nursing school to keep my clean cut appearance for Chuck's mom, Yvonne. I was not the first one up because I could smell the aroma of fresh baked biscuits I undressed and placed my wig on the hot water heater since there was no counter around the sink. I quickly bathed and dressed. I smelled a strange burning smell. As I reached over to grab my wig it had fallen down by the flame and caught on fire! Panicking I picked it up and placed it in the sink. "Oh my Goodness, what am I going do?" I screamed out loud. My hair was so frizzy from the humidity. I could not open the window to air out the bathroom. I had no choice but to call Chuck who had already taken Ricky and joined his family in the kitchen.

"Chuck help me, please!" He could tell the desperateness in my voice. He came quickly and opened the window when he saw the smoke.

"How did that happen?"

"I put my wig on the hot water heater and it fell and caught on fire."

"That wasn't too smart." His tone made me cry. "I am sorry, but look at me. I didn't even bring my Dippity Doo! I am so embarrassed what I am going to do? Can you find me a rubber band I will just put it into a bun." Chuck went to tell his mom of my accident. He returned with a rubber band.

Meek and embarrassed, I joined the family for breakfast. The only good thing was my introduction to the cheese biscuit. It had to be the best thing I had ever eaten for breakfast. Chuck's mom said without much conversation "Charles have Marion get into the car. I am taking her to the hair dresser, my treat." I did as I was told. I looked over and saw a twinkle in his dad's eyes. He looked like he was avoiding the urge to burst into laughter. I explained to my mother-in-law how Charles wanted me to look perfect. I was so embarrassed that I kept rattling on. When we arrived at the beauty shop she informed the hair dresser to put my hair up. Upon completion I looked like I was ready for the prom with a sixties type up do. Chuck's Mom said, "Much better. At least you won't be embarrassed." I made my grand entrance into the house. Chuck smiled right away.

"Is that you? You look real nice." Chuck's dad snickered, "Yes, you do. That was quite an experience. Welcome to the family." The ice was finally broken. His quiet little grandmother pulled me aside only to say, "The best time of my life was spent with a Catholic boy!"

My in laws informed us that they would be looking at land in Florida and most likely retire there. I did leave there feeling part of the family. Family was so important to us. Chuck received orders to Puerto Rico. This excited us because Dad was retiring and leaving Warner Robins anyway and they were moving back to Massachusetts. We found out that we would have base housing because we had a child. Our unit would be all furnished. It was so hard to say good bye but we knew it was our turn to travel.

Chapter 9

We arrived at Ramey Air Force Base in Puerto Rico. The ocean surrounded the base. Everywhere there were palm trees. Our sponsor greeted us and took us to temporary lodging. He was friendly and obviously loved this assignment. In three days we were processed in.

Moving in to our tropical home was exciting. It was a duplex across the street from the ocean. In front of our unit sat a huge banana tree with bananas dangling. Our sponsor said they made great plantations. We had no idea what that was but it sounded interesting. The inside had cold brown tile floors, no glass windows just shutters, and all new appliances. I knew it would be a challenge to make this home.

In just a week, we discovered all sorts of strange things. The banana tree sheltered a tarantula spider. Rats ran through the shutters. Our neighbors were alcoholics. Best of all a giant lizard laid baby lizards in the back yard. Little geckoes ran through out the house. Ricky had to sleep under a mosquito net. I just kept reminding myself how Mom said it was an adventure each time she moved. There was no television until evening. I was lonesome And while Rick napped, I managed to read sixty romance novels.

Chuck came home one evening and asked, "Can I invite this nice guy named Ken to dinner? He is a newly wed and they have no children. So they don't qualify for base housing. He is just so home sick."

"Of course you can. I will make spaghetti and meatballs." The next evening Chuck came in with his buddy. "Marion, this is Kenny."

"Hi Kenny, love your name that is my brothers name too. Hope you are hungry."

Chuck interjected, "We are starved!"

"Good let's eat." I put Ricky in his highchair and we had a great meal. It was so nice to have company. After dinner Chuck and Ken both played with Ricky. After putting Ricky to sleep, I joined them in conversation. "Kenny. You must be homesick."

Kenny replied, "I miss my wife Becky so much!" His eyes misted up showing his true emotions. We said goodnight and he walked back to the barracks.

"Marion what do you think if we invite Kenny and his wife to stay with us until they find a place off base?"

"Are we allowed to do that? I sure like him but what if we don't like his wife." After thinking some more, I went on, "He breaks my heart. We do have three bedrooms. I would love the company too. If it is legal we can do it."

"I knew you would say that. I told him I was going to ask you."

"What would you have done if I said *no* Smarty Pants?"

Chuck laughed, "I will tell him tomorrow after I talk to the first sergeant."

"Okay, well first, let's get some sleep."

Three weeks later Kenny and Becky moved in. I loved Becky from the start. It was like having family. I realized the only way to survive military life was to make your friends your family. We played pinochle every night. They adored Ricky. After multiple tries, we finally got the bacon to Becky's satisfaction: nice and crispy. We did a lot of laughing. Chuck and I grew up in the military. Waiting in long lines and finding unlabeled canned goods were not shocking.

One evening we decided to barbeque. Our neighbor, Pat, was rather a large woman and had passed out in the doorway from too much Rum. Rum was only a dollar a bottle. Her tiny little dog finished her drink and came running over and was walking crooked until he passed out. We felt like we were watching a live episode of our favorite 70's show, *Laugh In*.

Becky and Ken eventually found a cute little house right off the base. We actually missed them when they moved out. Chuck's 21st birthday was approaching. I managed to purchase a small motorcycle from one of his work buddies so Chuck could get around the base and Ricky and I could use the car. I had everyone we knew come over for a surprise party. I baked him a cake and drew a motorcycle on it. The guys put me on the bike and pushed it into the house. The look on his face was worth all the effort.

We heard rumor of Ramey Air force Base closing down. Not soon enough for me, though. Chuck got temporary orders to Warner Robins Air Force Base and left me there, alone; this was the part of the military life that I hated. While he was gone, Ricky took his first steps. He also got very ill with flu-like symptoms. One night he had soiled his bed and I moved him into my room into the playpen beside me. I was so exhausted from getting up all night long that I had fallen into a deep sleep. Our field phone rang in the middle of the night and it woke me right up. I hoarsely managed a, "Hello?"

"Marion, wake Ricky up. Roll him over now!"

Frantically I rolled my sweet baby over and he was turning blue. He had choked on his vomit. I cleaned his mouth and put him on my shoulder as he gasped for air and began to cry. The cries were music to my ears. I picked up the phone and questioned Mom, "How did you know and how did you get through to me on this field phone?"

"Oh I heard him cry. He is going to be fine. I just kept seeing it over and over in my mind. I knew something was wrong. Thank God, not me."

"I love you Mom. I gotta go. I will stay awake until he is all better! Bye bye!"

I was awake all night and day until Ricky was well. I was overjoyed when Chuck was coming home. I drove to the terminal to pick him up. I saw his plane land and they disembarked. When he saw us I whispered to Ricky, "There is your Daddy go walk to him."

Chuck saw him and fell to the ground stretching out his arms and started to cry. Ricky went right into his arms. At that moment I stopped and thanked God for all my blessings.

"Chuck it was so hard being without you. I hope we never have to be apart while we are here again."

"I didn't want to tell you this yet but next month they are sending us to Ecuador on a mapping mission for one month."

"You mean you will be in South America for a month and I will be stuck here, again?" I wanted to cry.

"Don't let it ruin our night," he coaxed.

"I won't but I want to go home and visit Mom and Dad, even if it means eating hot dogs for a month!"

"Okay I will see what we can do." Chuck kept his promise and bought us tickets to fly to Boston. He even purchased a ticket for the dog. Being able to go see my family made the separation much easier.

My destination was Billerica, Massachusetts. First I had to fly a four passenger plane through the mountains of San Juan. This was quite a feat with a baby and dog. Finding the gate was difficult all alone. I dropped the diaper bag and everything fell out. An obnoxious well dressed lady voiced her opinion, "You should not be traveling with a baby." I started to cry but refrained from telling her that my husband is defending our country. I promised myself never to be like her. I pulled my self together and headed for the gate.

Reaching our destination I felt very proud of myself. Dad got my luggage and I went to fetch Scooby. When I couldn't find him, I was informed that in our layover in New York City, they had accidently unloaded Scooby. The airlines promised to deliver him to Boston.

My family was thrilled to see Ricky. It was so wonderful to be with all of them again. Chuck wrote letters and called. He had fallen in love with a little shoeshine boy and wished we could adopt him. He flew a lot of miles mapping the entire country.

Retuning to Puerto Rico we had orders waiting, assigning us to Biloxi, Mississippi. While Ricky might have been born there, we never wanted to live there. But, it became more exciting when Becky and Ken were assigned there also. Chuck checked it out on the map and found his folk's home in Florida was only four hours away. After a short but long nine months, we prepared for our next journey.

Chapter 10

We arrived at Kessler Air Force Base. Cost of living was very low but we had no furniture. We found a little apartment and bought a recliner. We slept on the floor but at least Ricky had his crib. When Chuck re-enlisted, we were able to purchase a couch and table. Once a month we traveled to our in-laws home in Chipley, Florida. My relationship with them bloomed. His dad and I went in circles over religion. He loved to tease me and challenge me with deep questions like: "Marion, why do you tell your sins to a priest and not to Jesus?" My reply was simple: "Well the priest is like a phone operator straight to Jesus who tries to assist us with our problems and forgives us like Jesus would." The questions never stopped. "Marion, why is Jesus still on your cross? He has risen!" "Well it is to remind us of his suffering and how much he loves us." I would diligently respond. We grew to have mutual respect when it came to religion.

His sense of humor, on the other hand, took time to understand. He knew I loved animals. One visit he sent me out to the barn to pick out a bunny from his rabbit cages. I picked the cutest one I could find. I knew Ricky would love having him at home. Chuck's mom was busy in the kitchen so I kept Ricky outside, out of the way, playing until dinner was ready. He loved all the land to roam. They had a little fish pond that we loved to walk to. Both parents grew up on a farm and had green thumbs. They planted an acre size garden. There were rows of vegetables like: squash, green beans, okra and much more. For the first time, I was introduced to butter beans and okra. At that point, they were living in a double wide trailer while building their home. Everything was so green on their land. Chuck called us in saying, "It is time to wash up. Dinner is ready!"

We sat around the dinner table with his sister Belinda and little brother Dennis. His older brother, Donald, lived in North Carolina. His parents came to the table with a huge platter of fried chicken that smelled so good.

I blurted out, "I love fried chicken!"

Chuck's dad, Joseph, quickly responded, "Well Marion you start first." Then he handed me the serving platter. Joseph said his beautiful blessing and I ravishingly started to eat.

My plate was empty and I had to share with them, "This is the best fried chicken I had ever eaten." The whole table burst into laughter.

Joseph announced, "Marion it's not fried chicken. It is fried rabbit. You picked it out yourself." I left the table in tears but Chuck followed and calmed me down. I did realize it would be a family joke forever.

We were thrilled to find a little house to rent with a yard for Ricky. It was nice because now his family could visit us too. On Christmas Eve, they brought a mess of fish they had caught to our house. I was used to turkey. Our little house worked for gatherings but that was about it. The landlord was my first introduction to a redneck. He kept a killer dog in the yard to keep school children away. That dog bit the head off a little puppy I had gotten for Ricky while Chuck was on another temporary top secret duty. When I would tell him things about the house, like how the oven door wouldn't shut, he told me to prop a chair in front of it. Dreadful things only seemed to happen when Chuck was away.

I was so thrilled when Chuck told me he had applied for cross training to be a computer operator. We were both tired of the constant separations. We knew it would be a much more lucrative job outside the military as well. "Marion, computers are the way of future!" Chuck was accepted into the cross training program and our next assignment sent us to Wichita Falls, Texas.

While the Texas heat was dry, I was relieved it lacked so much humidity. It was dusty, though and rendered few trees. We rented a little duplex.

Everyone else in Chuck's class lived on base. Our little duplex ended up as the gathering place for homework and eating. It felt like a little USO. Ricky got plenty of attention. One night I put a buffet out with meatball subs and chips. Chuck asked me to get some beer, too. The guys poured their beer in paper cups to enjoy with their subs. I had ample paper cups left from our trip to Texas. Ricky had been in the midst of potty training and we could not stop often enough so they were used in lieu of stopping when he had to go potty. One of Chuck's closest classmates, Swede, put his cup, half-full on the table so he could goof around in the living room making a human pyramid. Returning all hot and sweaty from the little work-out, he gulped down the rest of his beer only to run to the sink and spew it out in disgust. Ricky had taken one of the familiar cups and urinated into it and placed it on the table. Swede's mild manor personality allowed him to laugh with the rest of the classmates. He had great sense of humor.

Swede was tall and slender with blonde hair. He was such an asset to Chuck because of his great teaching abilities. He was patient and personally guided Chuck through the class. He already had a bachelor's degree but there were no slots available so he entered the service as a non-commissioned officer. He made the time fun by planning activities like eating out together. When two of the classmates fell in love and married, Swede helped plan the wedding in which we all took part. The class graduated and received orders. Chuck and Swede both had orders to Omaha, Nebraska.

I loved the city of Omaha. We found such a nice townhome to rent. We quickly fell in love with the neighbors. I had accepted the fact that Ricky was our miracle and there would be no more children unless we adopted. But, all I could focus on was that adoptions cost so much money.

One night, Chuck took me out on New Years Eve dancing. He knew I wanted more children. I was feeling a little down. He had bought me a beautiful green gown. At midnight he whispered in my ear, "I think we will have a miracle this year I feel it. We are going to have a big family." I wanted to save money for adoption so I had sold all our baby items and went to work for a travelling nurse's association. I knew it was the only way to make a miracle. I cooked often for all of our friends and stayed so busy. I did notice I was gaining a little weight. One morning I told Chuck to place his hand on my tummy and feel how strong the gas was rolling in my stomach.

"Marion that is not normal you need to go to the clinic." I made an appointment. The diagnosis was a joyful shock. I quickly drove home to tell Chuck. "Honey, the doctor said that I am five months pregnant!"

"How can that be?"

"Well Honey, you know how babies are born, well it must have been that horrible snow storm when you came back to bed frozen after walking to get Ricky some milk and I had to warm you up!" I laughed, knowing he meant how I could be pregnant again with all my complications . . . but we were so happy we decided not to question this new blessing.

Along with the diagnosis came restrictions: no steps, no lifting, and minimal weight gain. That presented a major problem. I knew this was important to follow because my hips and back could get injured. Well into the 6th month, the baby sat on a nerve that caused me to drag my left leg. All the bedrooms were up a long flight of steps. We decided to try and rent a one level house but everything was out of our price range. We were so grateful to Swede because when he heard our news he offered to share our house with us and rent a room. We were blessed to have such a caring friend.

We found a house for rent in a wonderful neighborhood. It had three bedrooms. The street was lined with mature trees. Across the street lived an older Italian couple, Ross and Rose. They adopted all of us. Rose was a little woman but quite heavy. Ross was a city bus driver. They had one child. Rose cooked all day long. We loved it when we were invited to dinner to eat her amazing breads and pastas.

By the end of my pregnancy, our name came up on the base housing list. It would save us so much money and we were relieved that it was a one level house. Chuck's folks came to visit after we were settled. They were so excited to have brought up some fresh vegetables in a cooler and a treat.

"Marion, you go in the kitchen and put the things in the cooler away." Chuck's dad ordered. I thought he was being a bit bossy, but I did as I was told. I went into the kitchen and opened the cooler. Then I screamed! In that cooler was a skinned coiled rattle snake!

Everyone but I burst into laughter.

"Marion I caught that in my hard. I brought it for supper," He boasted.

"I am not cooking rattlesnake and my boys are not eating that!"

They cooked snake and my boys did eat it but I easily resisted. We enjoyed their visit. Joseph liked to tease me. I did have to take my gold crucifix off the wall in the guest room so Yvonne could sleep. Also, so I wouldn't have to argue that I knew Christ had risen!

Ryan was here before we knew it. The obstetrician performing the cesarean was fascinated that I carried a baby almost full term.

He asked me "When I close you up would you like me to make you a bellybutton?"

Excitedly, I replied, "I would love it!" The c-section went smoothly. I was put to sleep and woke up to Chuck telling me that we had a beautiful baby girl. They brought our precious baby in only for us to soon reveal that we actually had a baby boy. I was joyful and felt so guilty that I was upset when the doctor admitted he forgot to make me a bellybutton. The city shared our joy as well. They printed an article that our baby boy was born to a sergeant that was born at the same hospital twenty five years ago. Chuck's parents were stationed there in 1952. During my pregnancy, I walked to and attended a church named, *Saint Ryan's*. This miracle from God could only be named Ryan. Chuck was right we did have a miracle!

Chapter 11

My miracle kept me wrapped up in my own little world of joy. I was soon caught off guard by Chuck's lack of enthusiasm. I knew he was sad that his parents thought we did not need another child yet. I tried to convince him they were just overly concerned. After my parents came out to see the baby, Chuck's temperament had changed for the worse.

He acted as if he had the weight of the world on his shoulders. Christmas was a burden to him instead of a joy. I was trying not to let his odd behavior kill my joy and just put it out of mind. The holidays ended but Chuck's moods worsened.

One afternoon I received a call from the first sergeant. Chuck broke down at work. He checked himself into the hospital for depression. I felt overwhelmed with different emotions like guilt and anger. I called his mother and she flew out to visit him after the doctor requested it. Yvonne and I both met with the doctor. We realized that Chuck suffered from anxiety. It was more than depression; he had major concerns about our family. He was released after just a couple of days. He was ordered to take relaxation and music therapy. Chuck had to learn to express his feelings more. For instance, I never appreciated how much he liked country music. We purchased records that he liked. I found out he never minded at all that I did not have a bellybutton; but he did mind that I had birth defects. He felt he would have to always work hard to provide for me and two children. While I loved being at home with my children, I decided to go to work. I was angry that I had to change my life. I vowed to myself that I would never be a burden to anyone again.

Not being a burden was a hard job. I knew my white knight fell off his horse. I did not want to be angry. I wanted to make him as happy as I was and just love him. So, I endeavored out in search of a job. First, I had to find a sitter. My neighbor recommended a doctor's wife in the base housing area. I found work at a pizza place.

Ricky was in kindergarten and adjusted fine. Ryan was irregular and a little fussy. We all tried to adjust. The extra income took a financial burden away from Chuck. The kindergarten had an early release one day while I was scheduled to work so I arranged for Ricky to go to the babysitter. Chuck took off work early to pick them up and found about ten other children asleep in the living room with Ryan. Ricky was the only child awake. Chuck took them home and prepared dinner.

I was home in time for dinner. Chuck started to tell me his concerns.

"Marion, I thought Ryan didn't take a nap anymore. He was sound asleep with about ten other children when I picked him up."

"The sitter told me she watched only a few children from her church, and just occasionally!"

Ricky interrupted our conversation, "Mommy, is Ryan sick? Why does he have to take medicine to make him take a nap?"

Fear entered my thoughts, "Ryan is not on any medicine Ricky. Did you see the sitter give him medicine?"

"Yes Mommy, it was purple."

"Marion you need to call her now!" Chuck jumped up and demanded.

Immediately I called the sitter. She light-heartedly informed me, "It's nothing at all! I only gave him a teaspoon of Benadryl. On Wednesday I watch all the church kids and it puts them right to sleep." "In fact," She persisted, "My husband writes me the prescription."

I discovered a voice that I never knew I had. "That is not okay! Had you given that medication to Ricky he would be in the hospital. He is allergic to Benadryl. We will no longer need your services!" I hung up so angrily but proud of myself for voicing my concerns.

"Chuck I did not have children to have them abused! Now I know why parents want quality childcare!'

"Marion I will report this. Let's just watch our own kids. Why don't you try and work the night shift."

That is what we did. I worked nights and tips were better anyway. I brought the boys to work with me and Chuck picked them up. It was a different life than I imagined but it worked.

The manager at the restaurant owned a hotel and asked me to work the evening shift there. The money was good but we just didn't have enough time together. I was thrilled when Chuck came home and said we had orders for Hawaii.

Chapter 12

Traveling to Hickam Air Force Base was like a vacation. The base temporary quarters were full so we got to spend two weeks at a hotel. The cost of living was extremely high so we were thrilled that we got base housing. It was modern and had air conditioning. The first year was so exciting. We traveled around the island like tourists. Just like in Puerto Rico, Chuck brought a young man home named Ken. He instantly became part of our family. We threw him his 21st birthday party. Life got even more fun.

Back home in Boston, Ruthie had met and married a wonderful man named Bob. He had joined the service and unfortunately got stationed in Korea. There was no housing and they discouraged any family to join their spouse. Ruthie decided to come stay with us.

I had volunteered at the base gym to watch children while their mom's exercised. One of the participants loved how I interacted with the children. She offered me a position at her preschool in Pearl Harbor. I loved working there and I could take Ryan with me. Ruthie volunteered and came to work with me. We enjoyed the children so much. It was quite a different culture. Ruthie wanted to learn more about the culture and enrolled in King Kamahi's school. She even learned to hula. During the evenings, she curled up with my children.

Ryan, at the tender age of four, had formed a special bond with his Aunt Ruthie. They both looked so much alike. They had brilliant blue eyes and sandy brown, natural wavy, thick hair. In our off time, we went to the beach which was located right on the base. Ruthie had become my best friend; we wore bathing suits with skirts and thought we looked like old ladies. I suggested we swim by the docks one afternoon. Ruthie ran right into the water with Ryan by her side. I followed behind and was startled by Ruthie's scream "There are big fish in here."

"Don't worry just open your legs and let them swim by."

I did the same. The fish seemed to multiply.

"Ruthie I think these are the fish Chuck catches all the time so I think they are fine. I think we should find another part of the beach to swim, though!"

"I am with you. Let's get out of here!"

We got out of the water and found clear waters. A man approached us and told us we were swimming with hammerhead sharks. They liked to hang by the dock.

"Oh my goodness you took me into shark infested waters!" Ruthie was done swimming for the day. We laughed all the way home but I knew I would never hear the end of that.

Time with Ruthie ended much too quickly. Ruthie missed her husband tremendously. She was so brave and decided to join him in Korea and live off base. They found out she could go on base everyday and volunteer at the hospital while Bob worked. The house would seem so empty with out her. Chuck was always gone. Even with me working he still felt the needed to work part time. We put Ruthie on a plane to Korea. Ryan cried that night at bedtime. I told him Ruthie was family and we would see her again. She had already told him how Uncle Bobby was so lonesome. He seemed to understand.

I had hoped that with the house to ourselves Chuck would find more time to do things with us. The little preschool and the kids kept me busy. I got discouraged when Chuck started playing tennis at his lunch hour with the crew at work. He had formed a tight bond with the men he worked with. He was the only one married. Hopefully I didn't make him feel like he had a ball and chain attached to him. I felt he was restless. The boys started to get on his nerves and there were other little signs. I missed him and yet he was my husband living in the same house. I needed something more. My boss pulled me aside saying she needed a summer camp director and wanted me to have that position. I told her I did not have the money to get the education that the position required. She promised to get back to me.

I could not think of any way to go to school. I felt honored that she had so much confidence in me. Summer was along way off. We received a call from Swede saying he was coming for a three week visit. It was such a pleasant distraction. Showing him around the island was entertaining. We were amazed that Swede already knew our friend Ken.

I loved going to the beaches and Honolulu in the evening. Swede's visit was followed by a short visit from Chuck's parents. I loved their visit because Chuck stayed home. Chuck's mother was very much against drinking liquor. Her father would get very drunk and take her to the carnival forcing her to ride the rides until she vomited. We had already bought them tickets for a luau which included pina-coladas. We ordered their drinks virgin and took a picture of them toasting. Chuck could not believe how much they laughed even when we threatened to mail the photo to their pastor.

The visits stopped and our daily routine returned. Ken seemed to recognize the stress between Chuck and me. One evening he came over with a wonderful gift for us. He purchased two tickets and hotel reservations to the Island of Maui for three days. He was such a real friend. It was just what we needed. We arranged for my friend and her husband to watch the boys for our trip.

Maui was paradise. It was not congested like Oahu. Palm trees blew with the island winds, called Trade Winds and the beach waters were tinted with turquoise. Ken had even rented us a car.

We climbed into our little love bug wearing flip flops. Chuck had on cut offs and I wore a colorful moo moo. We had a map and went hunting for our motel. We traveled along the beach road finding the address of a five star hotel.

"Chuck, wow, that's it over there! That can't be right. We can't get out of the car the way we are dressed!"

"We are tourists and no one knows us! It is a bit intimidating!"

A bellhop came to open the door dressed in a white outfit and gold cape.

"This is fancier than the Hilton I had worked at part-time!" Chuck exclaimed. We walked to the front desk thinking we were at the wrong hotel. Sure enough we had a room reservation. The bell hop escorted us to the room. When we entered the room our jaws dropped open. It was sheer elegance from the tropical décor to the views. From the balcony we could see a large hot tub and pool overlooking the ocean. On the end table by the bed was a large pineapple wrapped in yellow cellophane. The card read: *Have a wonderful time! Love, Ken.*

"Chuck can you believe this? He has such a big heart!"

"No I can't. I want to have a wonderful romantic weekend!"

"Me too! You know Ken has become family to us and I think he is worried we might not be getting along so well."

"Let's try harder."

Chuck leaned over to kiss me and start our romantic getaway. It wasn't a long kiss because his hunger pangs took over, "We need to eat!"

"I bet the restaurant here is fabulous," I suggested.

"Well that is not going to happen! Look at the menu prices!"

"Whoa, I am not that hungry."

"We can drive around and find something."

We did drive and found a little Hawaiian burger shack. We giggled all the way back to the hotel. The rest of the weekend was like out of the movies. We drove around the island and got lost. Chuck stopped and drank guava juice from Island children selling it at stands. We ate pineapple and Maui potato chips in our room. We soaked in the hot tubs with other tourists bragging about their last trip to Acapulco. Chuck joined in saying this was much nicer: as if we had ever vacationed in Acapulco! We did not want the weekend to end. There we found laughter again and romance. I just prayed to God that we could keep our love alive.

I had come to realize marriage is hard work. Chuck was back at his awful schedule and I was back at work. The director approached me once again. "Marion I will pay for you to attend the University of Hawaii. There is a program that will help you become qualified. It is only two evenings a week," She explained. I was so excited I couldn't wait to tell Chuck.

That evening I stayed up until he came home, after midnight.

"Honey, I have some wonderful news!"

"What? It must be important for you to stay up this late."

"My boss is paying for me to attend the University. The course is only two nights a week."

"Why would you want to go to school? I don't even have a college education!"

"If I had a better paying job you wouldn't have to work so much!"

"I like working!"

"I know you do but you are gone so much!"

"We can make it work."

"I can't stay home two nights a week watching the kids."

"Chuck, I really want to do this."

"It just won't work! Now I need to get some sleep!"

I felt so defeated knowing that I was closing a door that was opened just for me.

My boss had no choice but to advertise the position in the paper. Chuck was aware that he had disappointed me and took it out on the boys. It got to the point that I was glad he had so many reasons to leave. A director was found for the school. She had moved here from Chicago. My boss asked me to help her get settled and assist her. This was difficult because she had a position I wanted.

We picked her up at the airport and took her to a hotel. She was short and walked with a limp. I did not find her too attractive. Chuck always loved to help people and said he would help her move.

We took her apartment hunting. Chuck helped move around some heavy things in the apartment. I had her over to dinner one night when Chuck said he would be home. The conversation turned all about her and my plan of making her feel at home had backfired. She boasted all about her accomplishments and education. At the end of the night, she only thanked Chuck for helping her. I was so glad when she left. Chuck was quick to say, "I am glad we helped her. She is really nice. She must be pretty smart to have two degrees!"

"I don't care for her much. I am smart enough to go to college too."

"If we didn't have kids maybe you could handle going to college. I am going upstairs to get a shower."

Needless to say I was furious to be dismissed so lightly. I went into the front room when the phone rang. I picked up the phone and Chuck had already answered it. It was my new director and I could not believe what I was hearing, "Chuck I am so glad you answered the phone. I wanted to personally thank you for all your help. Could I buy you a drink this weekend?"

Chuck replied, "No thanks I have to work. We did not mind helping you at all." She persisted, "Anytime you want that drink give me a call!" How was I going to work with a woman like that! Upstairs I went to confront my husband.

"Chuck what was that phone call all about?"

"She was just trying to be nice. You are being jealous! My guy friends and you talk all the time."

"I don't invite them out for a drink. Besides they are both our friends. We just met this bimbo!"

"Don't worry I am not going to have a drink with her!" I was so confused and sad. I had to find a way to bring our romance back into our marriage again but Chuck was so uptight. I wanted to hear him laugh again, too.

A carnival was setting up on the base. I asked Ken if he could watch the boys. I told him how our first date was at the carnival and how Chuck had spent his paycheck trying to win me a teddy bear.

Ken came over and was there when Chuck came home.

I blurted out, "We were going on a date!"

"A date? I finally have a night off. I am pretty tired!"

"Come on we don't have to stay long. It will be fun."

I ran upstairs to freshen up thinking he would follow. He still had not come upstairs so I went down to speed him up. He was in the living room offering Ken money to take me to the carnival.

I was heart broken and burst into tears, "Ken you can go. I am sorry. No one has to take me anywhere!" Ken uncomfortably left.

"Chuck I know you work hard but I love spending time with you. I can not force you to be with me."

"I am just tired that's all. I am not going to discuss this with you. You are being silly."

I took the car keys and left. I drove to the carnival and watched all the people out having fun. There were families and lovers and teenagers all enjoying the evening. I missed my husband. I knew it was time to talk. I had read a poem earlier in the day. It read something about: *if you love it set it free and it will come back to you.* I sure hope it would never come to that. I went back home to put the kids to bed. I could hear Chuck screaming at the boys when I walked in the door. He was disgusted that Ricky had not made his bed properly. "You should be able to drop a quarter on the mattress and it should bounce!"

He shoved him in the hall and Ricky started to fall down the steps. Thank God I was there to catch him. I calmed the boys down and put them to bed. I went into the bedroom and Chuck was crying. "Marion I was so angry I could have hurt our son. I am so sorry."

"Chuck it is Ricky you need to apologize to! You seem so unhappy and uptight. I am also becoming someone I don't like. We have to talk because I think I might have to leave Hawaii."

"You don't have to leave. I do love you!"

"I know you do. I am not making you happy though. I am having horrible feelings of inadequacies."

"Like what?"

"Women go around half dressed on this island and even in our neighborhood! Sometimes I think you may want to see what it would be like with someone else; maybe someone with a bellybutton and no scars."

He started to cry again. I thought he would deny what I was saying. Instead, he confirmed it.

"Marion I do wonder what it would be like. I am sorry you were my first and only."

I felt like a dagger was just slammed into my heart. I knew then I had to let him go.

"Chuck I am so tired. I want to go to college. I want to make you happy. Right now I can't do either. Tomorrow I am going to call Mom and see if I can move home. This will give us both more time to figure out what we want. You can enjoy the rest of your time here in Hawaii without us. I will always be in love with you. Please help me do this."

He kept crying and held me in his arms, but he never begged me to stay. The following day he called me from work and he had arranged travel arrangements to Boston. I called Mom and she encouraged me to come. In less than a week we were headed to the airport. Chuck told the boys to be good and that he loved them very much.

We had a long embrace and he kept apologizing and said he loved me too. I never had to be so strong in my whole life. I wanted to turn around and run back into his arms but I couldn't. Over and over the whole flight I kept saying to my self: *if you love him set him free*. Soon, we would be with my family.

Chapter 13

My family accepted us with open arms. They made a little attic apartment for me and the kids. The boys thought it was cool. We got them registered in school. I also registered them with the Boys Club. I found work at a corporate childcare in Chelmsford, the next town over. Things had changed, though. My father had a heart attack a few months before we had arrived. His medication caused mood swings and even unprovoked anger. I would try to keep the boys upstairs entertained and quiet. I would slip down and watch television in the evening. Dad would help cut out what ever curriculum project I was working on. I was invading their private time. Mom never said a word, but I felt it. Chuck wrote and sent money when he could. Then both boys caught the chicken pox, one right after the other. It was a new job and I could not take off yet. Mom nursed them every day. She was my angel but I could see the wear and tear. She had already raised six kids. I missed Chuck so much as the months slipped by. Ricky acted up so much. My sister Patty and I became so close. She would rescue me and have me to dinner and take me shopping. Ricky loved her husband Lew. One evening he refused to leave their home and he had to carry him out to the car. I knew he missed his Daddy. My sister Patty told me wonderful news. She and Lew were going to have a baby. She just glowed with her pregnancy. She was already pretty with her blonde hair, blue eyes and slight build. I was so happy for them. It reminded me of how happy Chuck and I were with Ricky. I never realized how much I did love him until I was away. I felt we were headed for divorce and some how I had to move on.

Mom was giving me a pep talk on my way to work. She was encouraging me to move on. "Marion you know you could be a director and then you would make more money."

"Mom I need to learn a whole lot more and go to school. I just don't know how to do that right now. I will look into it though. First I need to get a place of my own."

"Marion don't be ridiculous. You can not afford that now."

"I know but you can't keep taking care of me."

"Marion we are having a card party tonight. Dad is making those stuffed crabs you like. You can join us after the boys are in bed."

I did just that. By the time I got downstairs everyone was drinking and playing cards. Dad asked me to join one of the tables that was short a player, at the table sat one of my parent's friend's younger brother. He was handsome and shy. We had a great conversation while playing. I got up for a soda and asked if I could get him anything. He replied, "No I can get it myself." He jumped up and reached over me brushing my hand. All of a sudden he looked in my eyes and said "You are so sweet." Then he reached down and held my hand. The affection felt wonderful. I was starving for attention. We finished the game and I walked him to the door after everyone had left.

"Marion can I take you to a movie and see you again."

"Sure that would be fun."

He took me to the movies. We also went out to dinner one time. He was very shy and hard to converse with. But I loved his gentleness. We both did not want him to meet the boys. That would be too confusing for them. Come to find out he never wanted children. He would try if it meant having me in his life. That is when it hit me. I had only seen Chuck's faults. He was a man that did not shy away from his responsibilities. He worked three jobs to try and support us. It must have been so hard to be around all the single people at work in paradise. He did try. I recalled how he had rented a cabin at Bellow's Beach for Easter weekend just to please me. We had an Easter egg hunt on the beach. This man was not Chuck and never would be.

Our friend Swede was sad about the separation. He mailed me funny cards every week. One day, the card was different. He offered me a place to live if I wanted to start over in Washington D.C. It was definitely something to think about. I needed to become independent on my own though. I spent too much time listening to music day after day and dreaming it was really the only thing I could afford. At that moment, I was listening to *Islands in the Stream* by Barry Gibb. I was pleasantly interrupted by a phone call from Patty.

"Hey, Lew has to work next weekend let's get away and drive to Maine."

"Cool that would be so much fun. I know the boys will love that."

Saturday arrived before we knew it. I was disappointed in the weather. It was a bit gloomy. Patty guided me to the highway and we were on our way. We had only driven about thirty minutes when it started to lightly rain. Unexpectedly, out of the corner of my eye, I saw an old antique Studebaker car driving erratically. Patty yelled, "That car is sliding over the meridian. It is heading right in our direction." Unbelievably, I did not panic. In a few seconds, I realized I could not change lanes. It could not hit Patty's side of the car, she was pregnant or the rear by the boys. Whether it was right or not I turned where it would hit the drivers side. The impact was loud and we were all whipped around. The police came pretty quickly. The driver had just gotten his driver's license. His speed was just a little too fast for the wet roads. He was only sixteen. My car was still drivable as it only had body damage. Unharmed, we climbed back into the car.

"Patty, do you still want to go to Maine?"

"No, I want to go back to Mom's house and call Lew."

"Are you all right?"

She was rubbing her abdomen. "I think so. I am cramping a little. Maybe I should get checked out."

"Patty I am so sorry."

"Marion, it is not your fault."

I drove Patty straight to the emergency room. The boys were being so good. Lew came and met us there. Patty checked out fine. I was exhausted and relieved. I had a hard time sleeping that night. I kept thinking how we do not know what God's plan for us is. Our life could change in an instant. I thanked God for protecting Patty and the boys. I prayed very hard for her to have a healthy baby. I always thought too deeply when it was time to sleep anyway. I always felt I was on borrowed time. A fear of death would creep into my soul. That night, I felt my life needed to change.

I was glad to see Monday morning come. I needed a distraction and work would be the answer. I drove my regular route that morning. I was approaching the last intersection to work when a red truck ran the stop sign and broadsided me. My car rolled over into a ditch plunged me into the grass. I was oblivious to everything around me. I felt so cold.

The driver of the truck came down in the ditch. He helped me up.

"Miss, are you okay? I am so sorry. I have never done anything like this before. Are you sure you are okay?"

I just nodded to reassure him.

"Some one in the neighborhood must have called the police."

The police came and I managed to get them to call Dad. They told me the car was probably totaled. Dad gave me all the insurance information. Then he took me home.

I heard him call Patty to come sit with me while he ran some errands. Patty came over and made me a cup of tea. Her eyes were so sympathetic. I tried to thank her for my tea but the words would not come out. I wanted to share my thoughts with her. The most important question in my mind was *what is God trying to tell me?* No matter what I said it would not come out. I would start to stutter and then no voice. I could see the concern in Patty's face. "Marion two car accidents in one week are enough to put anyone in shock. I think we need to go to the hospital!" I drastically shook my head no. Patty put another blanket over me and wanted to call Mom. But she was taking my Grandmother shopping. She also called me in for work for the rest of that day and the next. When Mom came home I had fallen into a deep sleep. I felt good when I woke up but still, I couldn't talk.

I did not want anyone to fuss over me. Patty left and said she would be back in the morning. I gave her a hug. Mom put the boys to bed and I went up when they were sound asleep.

I woke up the next morning still unable to talk. Patty seemed angry.

"Marion you need to go to the hospital!"

I stuttered the word, "To-morr-ow"

Patty left the room abruptly. I could hear her on the phone but I did not know what she was saying. She returned to the room with a very determined look.

"You are not going to like what I did; but I had no choice. I called Chuck last night. He has a right to know what has happened to you. Marion he is at Logan Airport. He was so concerned and upset he had to see you."

I stuttered "Ch-uck is here?"

Tears rolled down my cheeks. I felt as if this might be what God wanted.

When I heard Dad's truck pull in the drive way I moved faster than I thought I could. He hugged me the moment I was at the door. We both began to sob uncontrollably. I looked up and saw Patty and Mom and Dad all crying. Chuck did not want to let go.

He whispered in my ear, "Are you okay?"

I whispered back, "I am now!"

I missed the smell of his Aqua Velva after shave and the sight of his pretty blue eyes. I missed his hugs.

"The boys will be so happy to see you." The words just flowed out of my mouth.

It was an amazing day. Chuck said he went on a military granted emergency leave. He was going to help me get a new car and find an apartment. That was the plan. The reunion with the boys was so healing for all of us. I noticed Mom and Dad made themselves scarce so we could have time together. I took the rest of the week off. Chuck slept on the couch that night. The next morning we woke with a list of things to do. First we got the boys to school.

I had a call from the insurance stating the car was totaled and they would be issuing a check. We got more for the car than I paid for it. Mom and Dad left again for the day.

"So are you ready to go?'

"I need to run upstairs and get my purse."

"I will come with you. I have never seen the attic before."

We both ran upstairs. I got my purse and he sat on the bed looking around the attic room.

"I thought the attic was more finished than this. I am so sorry you had to live like this. There is no ceiling and you don't have a bathroom up here."

I sat on the bed beside him. "Its okay we are used to it. I love my antique dresser."

He embraced me and apologized again. I reached up and kissed him gently and said, "It is okay." He bent down and kissed me passionately." In moments we made love with an awakened hunger that brought our bodies alive. It was different than ever before. I did not mean to blurt it out but as we laid with such satisfaction in each others arms I said, "Chuck I still love you."

"I still love you too. I have had sex that meant nothing with other woman. I am so stupid. It is best with you. It's great with you. Can you forgive me?" My mind should have been filled with turbulent emotions. All I felt was a sweet peace come over. I let him go but I think he knew that he had come back to me.

"Yes I can. We need to have a more intimate relationship. I hated you working all the time and resented everything. I did not appreciate all you did for us. I miss our home. I am sorry too. It was so hard to make you happy. Worst of all I felt inferior about my body."

"I wish I did not make you feel that way. I started to think it would be better with someone else but it wasn't. I want you to be proud of your body."

"Chuck I think God wanted me to set you free so we could appreciate each other."

We made love again. We had found a new intimacy. We quickly dressed and left the attic. I had just loved talking to him.

We went and sat at the kitchen table to talk more. "Marion I have orders to Colorado and I want you and the boys to come with me."

"I do not know anything about Colorado," but when I closed my eyes I projected a place of sunshine and peaceful harmony.

"I just do not know how to do it. We have so many bills. I am sorry I opened up an NCO Club charge account. With out your income it was too much to pay for everything."

"I want to be together, but there are some things that I need to happen, first."

"I know you want to go to school. If we get back together I promise I will help you. I promise I will be more patient with the boys. I know I get uptight. The military makes me crazy."

"I promise not to let your bad mood days ruin my day ever again. I want to spend my days happy. I will try to lift your spirits. If not I will just go about my day."

"Mom and Dad want to see me but there is no way I can afford to go to Florida."

"Chuck my check for four thousand dollars is in the mail. I have another paycheck from work too. We can all go to Florida and then fly to Colorado. I won't need to buy a car."

"I did not think about that. Are you sure you want to do this?"

"I am positive."

"I am going to call Mom and Dad." Chuck told his parents our plans. They talked a long time.

"Marion you are not going to believe what they said. They think God wants us together. I told them about finances. They want us to have a new beginning. They told me to bring our bills; they want to pay them off."

My family was overjoyed with our plans. Patty apologized again for interfering with my life. I quickly replied to her apology, "Patty your decision to call Chuck has been such a blessing. Thank you!"

Chuck and I thanked Mom and Dad for all they had done for us. I knew I would be forever grateful to them. Before we left for the train station Dad called the boys into the living room. He made a presentation of trophies he had made for the boys surviving Grandma and Grandpa Woodsie's house. I believe they were the ones that deserved the trophies. We cried and hugged at the train station as we departed for a new journey.

Chapter 14

Our visit to Florida was wonderful. Chuck's parents encouraged us to keep our marriage strong and shared advice. They did pay off our bills, expecting payments of ten dollars a month. It was such a blessing to have them care so much for our welfare. I really felt they had genuinely accepted me into their family and wanted us all together.

We flew to Colorado with such promise for a new beginning. The boys were as excited as we were. We found a little rancher to rent off base. Chuck was assigned to Cheyenne Mountain Air Force Base. He actually worked inside a mountain. It was so interesting. We spent weekends exploring beautiful sites like the majestic Garden of the Gods, Seven Falls and Old Colorado City. One weekend Chuck felt adventurous and we drove through the Mountains and explored a small mining town called Cripple Creek. We felt that we may have found a home! Neither of us had ever lived in the west. The trees weren't as abundant but the Mountain views from the entire city made up for that.

Shortly after we were settled in, I became ill with a gall bladder attack and required surgery. Healing was difficult because Chuck had used all his allowed military leave time. I counted on the boys helping to recover. Good health arrived just in time. We were able to move into base housing. It was nice to be in a neighborhood where the boys could have friends. The holidays were approaching and we got news that our friend Ken from Hawaii was out of the service and he had settled in Denver. Ken was excited that we were all reunited. We invited him down for Thanksgiving.

The turkey was in the oven. It felt so good to be together for the holidays. One thing I didn't miss about Hawaii was the lack of the four seasons. Chuck walked over to the dining room window and peeked out, "You have your four seasons, but fall didn't last long enough. It is snowing like cats and dogs!"

"Let's check the weather report."

We found out there were white-out conditions and the roads would be unsafe, if not already blocked off. We put off dinner for an hour and half. We knew Ken had already left Denver and was on his way. We thought he probably had to return home or stop.

"Marion, go ahead and serve dinner. I don't think he is going to make it."

Just as we pulled the turkey out of the oven we heard a knock on the door.

It was Ken. He looked like Frosty the Snowman.

Chuck embraced him, "How are you? How did you get that little Rx—7 through this storm? Come in and warm up!"

It was a joyful reunion. Chuck and I still believe in the military your friends are your family.

I was so pleased that God placed him back in our lives. Ryan was in school full time now so I taught preschool at a corporate preschool outside the base; I enjoyed my work so much. I was convinced this would be my career.

I was employed only a few months when the director asked me to interview for another director position in the company. I interviewed as she requested knowing I did not meet the education standards. Much to my surprise I was hired for the position. I would be issued a temporary license as long as I was in school. I had been granted a second chance. But, I loved my life. I was uncertain of whether or not I should make an issue over it or let it pass? I needed to talk to Chuck. I went home and made a wonderful dinner. Then I sent the boys upstairs to read.

"Chuck, I have some exciting news. We need to talk."

"Okay, I will turn the television off," curious, he clicked it off and said, "What's going on?"

"I interviewed for a director position and got it! I have to go to school in Denver. The University of the Rockies will let me go up to take a class and then five weeks later after I do all the home work I can test. I know you promised to help me go to college but if you don't want me to I will stay teaching preschool. You are more important to me than my education."

"I want you to do this. I don't mind watching the boys but we can't afford it."

"I called the credit union and they said I qualified for a student loan. We can afford payments; because my salary will double."

"You should try it then. I will help as much as possible."
"Thank you! I LOVE YOU!"

And, I did it. I enrolled in college. I shocked myself. I handled working full-time and school. Child development had become my passion. I absorbed information like a sponge and was able to apply it to my work. I applied my new gained knowledge with the boys also. Ricky was my wild child. I realized that I often bribed him to behave with McDonalds and when he was misbehaving I still took him to McDonalds out of convenience. I learned never to make an empty threat if I had not planned to follow through. I could not have done it with out my husband cooking dinner and spending time with the boys on Saturdays. In less than two years I finished my schooling and received my Colorado Director License.

With my license there was an increase in pay and we were able to buy our first house close to the childcare center. The center grew to maximum enrollment. One lady came in to enroll her daughters. She was attractive and tall with soft blond hair. I looked forward to her picking up the girls every evening. She always greeted them with a smile. Her daughters were my boys' age. Her name was Diana. She loved to talk as much as I did. We were amazed to find out that she and her husband knew Ken and Swede. In a short time we became great friends. Diana worked for the Olympic Center, her husband worked for a local mail order company. She was always bringing in free supplies for the center: which we desperately needed. Our circle of friends increased when Chuck brought home someone from work nicknamed Wes. Wes was 6'5 with thick, curly, dark hair. His sense of humor was amazing. It was outstanding how he could make Chuck relax and enjoy the moment. Wes and I shared Catholicism and the fact we projected short life spans for ourselves. He loved deep intelligent conversations which I thrived on.

I was tired from putting in long days without breaks. Our center had growing pains. I did not like working for such a large national company. A local childcare owner approached me and offered me a position in one of his centers. He informed me that I would receive free childcare for the boys and two hundred dollars a month increase than what I was already making. Chuck and I discussed it and both agreed it was the right move.

Working for my new boss was like a breath of fresh air. The days were longer with a refreshing two hour break in the middle of the day. The boys loved coming to my center after school. I was given the opportunity to manage in my own unique style. Mr. Smith had enlightened me with his business and marketing skills. He was not a micro-manager. I enjoyed creating my own menus. Planning summer activities for our camp was an exciting challenge. The boys looked forward to our summer camp.

Eventually, I had hired my own staff and created a wonderful bond with my staff. Mr. Smith planned monthly lunch meetings to instruct and guide all the directors. I never felt that I was going to work. Each day was delightful. I also wanted to contribute to our community. I volunteered for the March of Dimes. We did puppet shows and education visits to childcare centers. I became chairwoman for the mini walks and president for the Mountain Valley Chapter of March of Dimes. I always just wanted to appear normal. I always concealed my birth defects. A beautiful little red-headed toddler named Emily attended my childcare center. Emily had Down syndrome. Her mother was attentive and creative to encourage her development. She brought in her own playpen that had mirrors and toys all tied to it. Emily's mom reminded me of Mom. Mom would tie balloons on my feet as a toddler to encourage me to exercise my muscles by kicking. That allowed my muscles to strengthen which made walking easier after my surgery.

Mom flew out for our Mother's March campaign. She was honored to be part of this wonderful event. We picked her up at our little airport. She was dressed in a flamboyant purple hat with a matching purple coat. She unexpectedly asked "Where are the cameras?!" I think she was disappointed that we had to go to the cameras as opposed to them finding us. Together, we did radio and television talk shows. I found it so humorous that Mom was so shy on television. She did have the gift of gab but not in front of the camera. Our center grew to capacity. I speculated that Mr. Smith wanted to sell the childcare center. My heart had become awakened with the desire to meet the needs of all children. I desperately wanted to run my own childcare business. All I lacked was the funds. Eagerly, I shared my interest in our friend Ken and he wanted to provide the financial backing. I was unaware he even had any money for investment. I was delighted with his faith in me but I bore the burden of the possibility of letting him down.

We formed a corporation and went into business as *Little Einstein's Learning and Childcare Center.* The adventure was like a college education in business. The building laws changed. There were huge sex scandals in California which inevitably hiked the cost of insurance. Teachers were required to take training classes. My dream slowly became a financial nightmare but we kept drudging through it.

We were pleasantly distracted with the holidays approaching. A little girl that attended the preschool was in custody of foster parents because her mother had abandoned her. I had instantly fallen in love with this child. She was plain with a sweet smile. Chuck and I decided to try and adopt her. I spent numerous hours investigating the adoption process. I learned that we had to take classes at human services weekly, so we arranged the time. We needed a home where the child's room would be next to us. There was an endless amount of paper work, but Chuck was eager to take on that task.

With the entire daily tasks I faced, I still needed to think about Christmas presents. We always did the boys by putting them on layaway in September. The best way to describe Chuck's Christmas spirit was *Bah Humbug*! He dreaded shopping and decorating and putting up the tree. There was no surprising him because he always figured out his gifts. I was exhausted searching for the perfect gift. I entered my last store searching desperately.

A cluttered clearance table caught my attention. I frantically ransacked the items on display. There, I spotted the perfect gift. Folded in a large white box, lay the most realistic Santa suit that I had ever seen. It even had a matching beard and wig set. I had goose bumps as I purchased my treasure. I quickly ran home and hid it under our bed: not to be opened until Christmas Eve.

Our case worker informed us the adoption would not be considered because an out of state grandmother came forth to adopt her granddaughter. We were so disappointed and discouraged, but we found happiness in the fact that she did have someone to love her. The case worker told us to still turn in our journal and family photo album. We would be put on the list to foster adopt but it would be a long waiting period.

The day following Thanksgiving I needed a Santa to visit the center and kick off the season. I was shocked that Chuck volunteered so I let him wear the Santa Suit I had purchased by telling him just a little, white lie, "Chuck I rented this for you to wear." He believed my fib. He was a wonderful 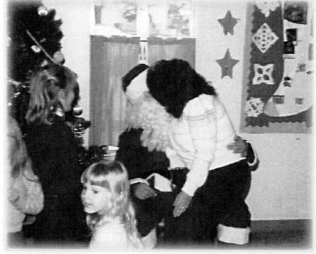 Santa with a robust "Ho Ho Ho"! I sat on his lap and whispered in his ear, "Thank you, I love you!" Then, I kissed Santa. One of the teachers snapped the photo. I cherished the picture so much that I placed it into our adoption journal before turning it in.

Chapter 15

We closed on our new house that we needed for adoption. Seeing the empty room made us sad. The house was fabulous. It had four large levels. The main level had a huge eat in kitchen, dining area and living room. The living room had a slated wall so that you could see the white brick fire place down in the family room. We kept reminding ourselves how God had blessed us with two sons when doctor's had insisted it was impossible. I was able to fill the lower level with an orange recliner and a Middle Eastern bar that had camels for bar stools. These strange conversational pieces were acquired from two different families that had gone bankrupt and couldn't pay their childcare bill. Legally they didn't have to do anything: but it relieved their guilt. Business was quite a complicated endeavor. One cold evening in early December we received a call from an enthusiastic caseworker rambling on, "I saw this picture of Mommy kissing Santa Claus and I realized immediately that you were the family to adopt these foster children. I promised their mom that I would find a special family. I believe you are it. Can we meet tomorrow?" Excited and anxious, we canceled our plans and made the appointment with the caseworker. He was a rather large, jovial man. He revealed that the children's parents were separated. Both parents suffered from drug and alcohol abuse. He portrayed the mom as loving her children so much that she wanted them to have a good home. I felt so much compassion for her. I could not imagine giving up our children. The caseworker appeared pleased to have chosen us. The only stipulation is the mother wanted to meet us and have a little Christmas with her children. We accepted all the conditions. Before we knew it we were on the porch of the receiving home holding hands before we knocked on the door. Chucks hand was quivering just like on our wedding day.

    The foster mom greeted us and guided us into the living room. On the couch sat a smiling redheaded girl with big brown eyes. It was love at first sight. I started a conversation with her asking her name. Giggling she replied, "I am Elisa Hope." I looked over at Chuck and saw him distracted by the cutest blonde haired boy with chubby cheeks and big brown eyes. He sweetly asked Chuck, "Will you be my Daddy too?" Chuck picked him up with tears of joy in his eyes and replied, "I sure hope so." We knew God had listened to our prayers yearning for a large family and fulfilled our prayers. We were disheartened over the large number of children in the receiving home. These children were not in their own home for the holidays. There were three Hispanic girls that looked like stepping stones. Their long black hair flowed to their waist. The foster mother of the receiving home said there were not enough foster homes available to place all the children over the holidays. Some children were put in foster care because of the financial stress over the holidays. Unexpectedly, we were able to take the children home that day with out the ritual of visitations.

    Chuck took two weeks of leave to help them adjust before having them come into the childcare. There was so much information revealed that we were unaware of. Their mom had placed them in the custody of a family with out the proper legal paper work. The family did not meet the qualifications for adoption. They only wanted to adopt Zachary, the blonde haired little boy.

    I could not imagine separating these two beautiful children. The bond between them was deeper than blood. Elisa took care of him like a little mother and she was only four years old. They played with each other joyfully. We went to the play room at the social service building. The children played while we met their birth mother. Michelle was beautiful with the same brown eyes of Elisa and Zachary. She explained that she had made a mistake of leaving her children to the other family. The kid's birth names were Brooke and Brandon. She requested that we change their names back and call them that. We both loved those names and agreed to do so. I shared with Michelle that Brooke was one of the names I had actually considered if I had a girl. I also shared that we could not have any more children. She asked if we would let Brooke's hair grow out. I knew we did not have to honor her desires but I wanted to alleviate as much pain as possible. How tragic to have so much love for your children that your addictions robs the ability to parent them. She asked one question that touched my soul, "Could you adopt me too?" We all laughed and cried.

She entered the visitation room with a large glass window. She had already placed Christmas presents under the tree for them. I know she created a very strong loving memory for them. Then, she hugged Brooke and Brandon good-bye with tears steaming down her cheek. It was a moment I would never forget. She gave us a gift that God gave her. I promised God that we would treasure our gift the rest of our lives.

We had to have Brooke and Brandon in our home for one year before we could legally adopt them. Then we would undergo scrutiny from home visits and therapy. Complications arose within the first few weeks. Their previous foster parents filed suit challenging their placement. Both families had to attend play therapy where a child psychologist would decide what was best for the children. My heart ached at the thought of possibly losing Brooke and Brandon. The previous family entered and we had to let the children go into the play area with them. Brandon gave them his heart wrenching, shy smile and went with them. Brooke froze, "Mom, are you coming in?"

"Brooke we will be in momentarily, I promise." She reluctantly entered the room with them.

It was finally our turn. Chuck got on the floor and played fire trucks with Brandon.

Brooke took my hand and said, "Mom let's play house. You are the kid and I am the Mom. You need to set the table. I am calling Diana over for coffee."

We relaxed so much in our play session that it passed quickly. The psychologist said that the report would be sent to our caseworker.

The next day the caseworker called me at work. "Mrs. Barnes the report specified that the children's best interest was to be adopted by you and your husband. She was quite amazed how quickly they had bonded with both of you. It was noted that Brooke role modeled you as well." The stress left my body and was replaced with sheer happiness. I couldn't wait to phone Chuck.

Now that things had started to fall in place we shared our tidings of joy with our parents. They both were pleased. Mom and Dad immediately called us back, "Marion we purchased tickets. We want to meet our new grandchildren! We will be there by Friday. It's just for a quick visit so we can be home for Christmas. This was an unexpected thrill. Diana had planned a big kid baby shower for me. Having Mom attend made the event even more special. Mom and Dad arrived and it eternally became my favorite holiday weekend of all time.

The baby shower was awesome. We received much needed clothes for Brooke and Brandon. At home they put on a fashion show. Mom and I felt we had Barbie and Ken life size dolls. That night after the kids were in bed, Mom and Dad played Santa Claus for an early Christmas day since they needed to be home before the actual Christmas holiday.

Brooke and Brandon giggled and laughed the whole weekend. Rick and Ryan played with them so much even with the age difference.

Our new family editions must have thought that life was one big celebration. Following Mom and Dad's departure, awaited Christmas Eve. After church we started our party.

I guided Chuck to our bedroom to privately give him the amazing Santa Suit.

He eagerly opened his gift, "Wow this looks like the suit I wore in the childcare."

"It is the same suit. I bought it for you. It's the suit that brought Brooke and Brandon to us."

'When should I wear it: while our friends are here or when they leave?"

"We should share Santa with everyone!"

It was a magical Christmas for all of us.

The year flew by with so much going on. It seemed smooth sailing until Brooke and Brandon's father located the company I worked for. One of my dear friends was the director at a different location. Their father tried to kidnap a blonde little girl and a red headed little boy from her center. Brooke and Brandon were with me. Luckily my friend intercepted and prevented a horrible mistake. He did not recognize his own children. He tried to stop the adoption; he probably saw it posted in the newspaper. I'll never forget how the judge asked him why he had wanted them back. He responded, "My wife will come back to me; if I could get the kids back."

The judge then asked, "Do you know their birthdays?"

He replied, "I can't remember."

The judge continued to batter him with questions about his children. We were not allowed to attend the hearing so we were thrilled that the caseworker revealed the hearing to us. The judge threw his request out of court. This turn of events meant we could finally set a date for the adoption. I was damaged by the turn of events. I would wake up in the middle of the night to make sure Brooke and Brandon were safely in their beds. Other nights I would be driving my car to rescue them and run over the predator.

Christmas was here once again. Chuck and I volunteered to play Mr. and Mrs. Santa Claus for the foster children's Christmas party. We even had our children help. I knew we had been spoiling our boys but this gathering of homeless children changed all of us. I was on stage beside Chuck. I was thrilled that my new Mrs. Claus outfit arrived in time. It was such a special gift from Chuck's mother. She sewed it and made a beautiful crisp white apron that topped it off perfectly. My mood quickly changed when a teenage boy sat on Santa's lap. He said, "Santa I am dying. I love music and I want a boom box so I can listen to music while I die." Santa had not promised anyone a gift until now. He wiped the tears out of his eyes and said, "Son, I promise you will have a boom box for Christmas." Chuck found someone in charge and then arranged for that young man to have his wish granted. We shared that story with our children and friends.

Thank goodness for our close friends. One morning our friend Wes called me at work to invite me to lunch. He said Chuck would join us later. I was thrilled that I had dressed up in a light gray suit. The children at the center were preparing for lunch when I heard a horn honk. I walked out to see Wes' car pull into the parking lot. Through the sun roof of his car a large Gumby poked out. He maneuvered out of his car wearing a giant Gumby doll hat. He had hot pink and green shorts on down to his knees and wore sandals. He was such a sight to see that I uncontrollably broke into loud laughter. I had to bring Gumby in to see all the children. I don't think the teachers appreciated how wound up we got them before their quiet time. It was a moment to be shared though. Even children have to break up their routine.

As mini-vacations, we would take the kids and with friends, get away on camping trips. Our camping trips were gathered around a fire at night where we shared stories. One particular campfire we were in deep conversation when we smelled rubber burning. One of my girlfriends did not even realize that her sandals were on fire. When we weren't gathering around campfires, we gathered at our home. Occasionally, Diana and I would talk everyone into going dancing. Diana was our dancing queen. I loved being around her because of her positive energy. I used only qualified sitters. I also had a lovely college girl that lived with us. She was in school to be a teacher and worked part time at the center. We unlisted our phone number and let everyone know the situation with the children. Our friends were a wonderful diversion.

Our friends joined us for the big adoption day on February 14, 1986. It was an astounding Valentines Day. The judge required each child to take the stand and he asked whether or not they want to be adopted.

Without hesitation, they both replied, "Yes."

The judge then asked, "Do you know what being adopted means?"

Brandon excitedly replied, "Yes I get to change my name to Barnes; I want to be 'Mr. T.' Barnes!" Laughter rang through out the courtroom. We celebrated with a big breakfast and later that evening a pizza party.

Months later into summer, as the childcare center bored more financial burdens, I had also become quite ill. Everything I ate went right through me. I had this problem slightly after my gall bladder attack but it was worsening. I avoided eating out. I could not understand what caused it and neither could the doctors. I started to only eat at night when I was close to the restroom. That only caused weight gain. One day I had to make a deposit for the March of Dimes at the bank and without warning, a yellow bile dribbled down my legs. I was so humiliated. I started becoming depressed. I was in such agony. I revealed my despair to Mom. She insisted I fly home and go to Beth Israel Hospital. We could not afford to all fly. Chuck drove with the boys. Brooke came with me. I made it special because it was her birthday week. Our dear friends Becky and Ken were our angels and let the guys stay over on route to Boston. I poured down medicine to bind me up for my flight. I was an outpatient for seven days as they ran a battery of tests. I was exhausted but felt rejuvenated at the diagnosis. I had an over bile production. All I needed to do was take a medication before going to bed every night. I had a new lease on life. I thank God that my mother insisted on me going to a specialist that was familiar with my history. I was anxious to get back to our childcare center.

Ken had stayed busy overseeing the center in my absence. I was ready now for fall enrollment and enjoying good health. I needed to focus on making our venture productive.

However, we soon learned that we had something more to celebrate. Chuck had received an isolated assignment to North Dakota. We had time before we left to prepare. I decided to sell the childcare center at a loss since the financial burdens were so severe. We merged back in with Mr. Smith's company. I was working at half salary to balance loan payments and for a moment, we weren't even sure we would be able to accompany Chuck in North Dakota. But when the news came, I was overjoyed to find out they had eight house quarters for families and we could get in one right away.

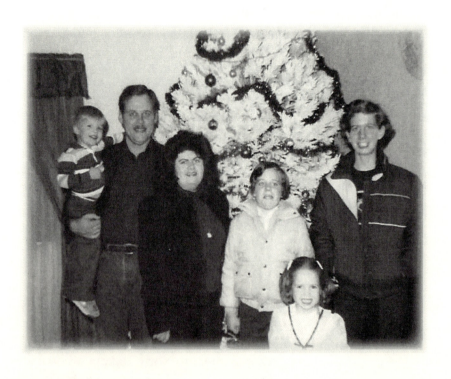

Chapter 16

It was agonizing saying good-bye to our dearest friends. Diana gave us the most enjoyable farewell party. I couldn't stop crying. They all understood how important it was to be together with our new family. Chuck and I loved having space away from the familiar grounds of their biological father to allow Brooke and Brandon to grow older and be safe. Nevertheless, I still feared them being taken away.

Once we arrived in North Dakota our fear vanished. We were twenty-five miles away from the nearest town. No one could find us, no matter hard they tried. We had an apartment sized unit. It was a shock after living in such a large home. I decorated it like a little country home. We could just hibernate for two years here. I thought it would be easy to find work but I was mistaken. We had to to get used to living on the small site, where as a base is a lot bigger.

Shortly after settling in, we were financially challenged because two thousand dollars was taken from our military pay from the IRS. Our accountant had made a terrible error. The law had stated that we were accountable. Things got tight. Luckily, there was not much to do. We all gathered in the base police station basement. It became a sort of recreation center. There was a large kitchen and games. Chuck even became a volunteer D.J. for dances. We were all allowed to use the base gym. I volunteered in a little town at a catholic preschool. In return, Brandon got to attend their private kindergarten. The public school was so small. It held grades first to twelve. Ricky had such a hard time adjusting. He was a more modern type than the local children. He, unfortunately, fell for the wrong girl and was attacked by another angry, out of control, student. I wanted to change his school to another little town. There was a contract for the military children to attend only one school. I requested a meeting with the school board and pleaded my case and motherly concerns. My request was granted to transfer. I was unable to volunteer at the catholic school but was referred to a childcare that hired me as a teacher's aid. I was so happy. I fell in love with the little town of Cavalier. The childcare board of directors said I was overqualified but I was just thankful to have a job. It appeared as if things would work. But, that thought was deceiving.

We had a change of command. The new commander was overbearing. And, of course, he moved in right across the street from us. The site gave each family a garden plot. We had the only dog. Her name was Candy. Even the young soldiers would come down and play with her. She followed me everywhere. If she was left outside, she would sit on the porch until we returned. We had been on site with our dog for eight months when Chuck was written up for Candy not being on a leash. We had Ricky's sixteenth birthday party at the basement of the police station. Everyone had their birthdays there, yet, we got written up for misuse of a government facility. I planned a field trip for the older children in our center to the site. We went through all the proper and required channels. But, Chuck was written up for not letting the commander know. The commander's wife started a group for women: *The Bored Wives Bunch*. It was scheduled to meet every Wednesday morning. I was unable to attend because I needed to work; with consequence, Chuck received a slap on the hand from his superior officer which was ordered by the base commander; this frustrated him greatly.

"Chuck I need to leave here before I ruin your career!"

"Marion I could not handle it here without you! You have done nothing wrong." He looked me in the eyes and reminded me, "We volunteer for Moral Welfare and Recreation. We volunteer and bring supplies up for the little store. We plan activities. Don't worry about my career." After careful thought, he continued, "Marion I know you are going to be upset because you're a USO girl at heart; but, the base commander just put out a letter stating that Christmas Eve and Day were to be family time, meaning no helping the soldiers here without their families because there will be no use of the facilities for gathering."

"Chuck how can she do that? What about all the young airmen and young officers in the barracks? They have no family here. That breaks my heart! Well no one can tell me what to do in my own home. I will set up a buffet and invite everyone over. It's Christmas! Is that okay with you? Will you get in trouble?"

"Marion I am already in trouble all the time, it will make no difference. There will probably be only ten guys left here that will not be able to go home. I will quietly get the word out."

We had a unique but extremely warm and wonderful Christmas Eve. I made a ham and turkey. We pushed our table up against the wall to clear space in our little quarters. Chuck played Santa and we sang Christmas carols. One young soldier brought over his guitar. Our kids gathered around him by the tree. That Christmas we were all family. When the holiday season came to an end, Chuck was written up for fraternizing with the officers. He told me not to let it ruin the memory of our Christmas.

The young couple that lived in the first quarters was going home for a summer vacation and asked us to watch their cat. Chuck was slightly allergic but Brooke was so excited he agreed to do it. The cat bit Chuck the first day so we all kept our distance from him. He was not the friendly cat they promised he would be. The following day some of the soldiers snuck into our backyard because Chuck was barbecuing. They all came in the house and played with the cantankerous cat. We had the cat one more day and he started to drool at the mouth and seemed sickly. Chuck took him to a vet down town. He came home white as a ghost. He said, "Oh my God Marion, they think the cat might have rabies and they have to test him. The only way they can test him is by cutting off his head!"

I panicked, "That cat bit you!"

"I know and they said that we should get shots."

"I guess we will just have to wait and see. We will just tell the kids the cat was so sick he died. Man I hate to tell our friends on vacation."

We were all petrified when the cat tested positive for rabies. This made it difficult to keep our fraternizing with the troops quiet, since they too had to get shots. Anyone that was in our unit or the cat owner's unit or had physical contact with someone who had played with the cat needed to receive rabies shots immediately. That was basically the whole site. There was not enough serum. They had to air vac some to the site. Doctors arrived to administer the series of seven shots: two in the bottom and five in the arm. It took about six weeks to complete. They made sheet walls for curtains to allow privacy. It even made the newspapers! Chuck survived the ordeal with no write ups though; we both looked forward to the end of our tour.

There was a small farming community right outside of the site. A wife of one of the farmers worked in the building with Chuck. She asked if we would be willing to coach a children's baseball league and if I would coach the T-ball league. We enjoyed coaching and it kept the children busy while the farmers harvested their crops. The community paid us five hundred dollars. We had an amazing time and our own children got to play as well. Chuck new I couldn't run the bases. He encouraged me by saying you can teach anything. Which I did and rather well after he taught me the rules of the game. That summer I flew home with Rick and Ryan for my brother George's wedding. My suitcase was lost but retrieved just in time. Then, unexpectedly, I got a call from the base commander. Chuck had fallen on a rock while fishing and had a serious infected blood clot. He said it was serious and that I needed to return home as soon as possible. He informed me that Brooke and Brandon were safe with neighbors but Chuck was in a hospital in Grand Forks. I was scared but returned as soon as possible. I worried dreadfully about Chuck. I panicked thinking of Brooke and Brandon not having either of us around with all the transitions in their young lives. Chuck's parents were on route to visit us along with his brother's family. When I got out to the site, Chuck's folks had brought Chuck home. I was told it was a serious infection and they had a hard time finding an antibiotic to work. My neighbor did a wonderful job telling the children that their visit was a little vacation. Brandon was a little scared, but survived. We had a nice visit with his family but were unable to do many things because Chuck was very weak. Because the summers in North Dakota were so hot and humid, we thought we were looking forward to cooler temperatures, little did we know those temperatures were 50 below.

Christmas came and it was the coldest Christmas, ever. Chuck volunteered to play Santa for our families stationed on site. We had also planned on sledding together before the party. It was twenty degrees below zero. I was pouring hot chocolate for the children when I looked up and saw my husband's sled sliding down wildly. In that same instant, he was thrown from his sled and hit a phone pole bending his body back like a horseshoe. I dropped the thermos and ran feeling weak from despair. I heard someone yell, "Call an ambulance!" Chuck was conscious. Amidst all the trepidation and fear, I admired how all the soldiers surrounding him took off their coats and laid them over him to prevent him from going into shock. We were all concerned because he could not feel his legs. The ambulance finally arrived to take him into town. I directed the kids to the car and we followed the ambulance. The small hospital was not equipped to care for Chuck and planned to transport him to the military hospital in Grand Forks, again, ninety miles away. Distressed, the kids and I went back to the site to get clothes and food for the journey. The base commander called saying he arranged temporary lodging for us. To make matters worse, the weather report said we were about to get bombarded by a strong snow storm.

Ricky and Ryan were concerned about who would be Santa Clause. I was in a daze and barely functioning. I did manage to tell them to pack up clothes. I told Ricky to gather snacks. I promised the children that we would celebrate Christmas when we returned back home. I managed to call my in-laws to tell them about the events. I was quivering at the thoughts flowing through my mind. I had to be functional and purposely did not ponder Chuck's condition. I felt blessed when Ricky took charge and told me to get in the car.

"Mom, the car is loaded and I am driving. You are too upset to drive. Get in the passenger side." I could not believe I allowed this with the impending snowstorm. Ricky had just acquired his driving license. His confidence and authority reminded me of his dad and I handed him over the keys. I could feel God's presence watching over us. The roads were atrocious but Ricky courageously maneuvered the vehicle safely to our destination. I checked into our reserved unit and the boys unpacked the car. I tucked Brooke and Brandon into bed and kissed them goodnight. I told the boys I would return as soon as I knew how Daddy was. The second I saw his face, the tears rolled down my cheeks. He could not stop saying, "I am so sorry I ruined Christmas."

I reassured him, "Everything is going to be all right. We will celebrate Christmas when you come home."

We were interrupted by the doctor, "Sergeant Barnes there is too much swelling in your back to know the extent of the damage. We will be able to tell more tomorrow.

As he left the room I stroked Chuck's wavy brown hair and wiped the tears off his cheeks.

"You would be so proud of your children. Ricky drove all the way here. He tried to fill your shoes. Ryan took charge of packing things up so patiently for Brooke and Brandon. Those kids did not flinch when I told them we will celebrate Christmas when you come home."

Visiting hours had ended and I needed to return to our children. I kissed Chuck goodnight, and said, "I will see you in the morning."

"Marion what if I never walk again?"

"Chuck it will all be fine. We will find everything out in the morning." I tried my hardest to conceal my dreaded fear that he may not be able to walk. I knew I could not dwell on that. I had to put my faith in God. I could not wait to get back to the kids. I knocked on the door and Ryan opened it saying, "Merry Christmas." To my astonishment, Ryan was wearing his father's Santa suit. Together, they had pushed the little kitchen table against the wall to substitute for a Christmas tree. I was in such mental turmoil that I had not noticed they brought the holiday treats and my crock pot of Sloppy Joes. The little lodging smelled like home. I was so joyously flabbergasted when I saw Brooke and Brandon's presents under the tree like table.

I asked, "How and why did you do that?"

Ryan said, "Mom they still believe in Santa, we didn't want to spoil it for them."

Ricky added, "When you were on the phone to Grandma Barnes we pulled their presents out from under the tree. There wasn't room for ours but we can wait." I cried tears of joy and pride as we shared our little Christmas feast. This was not the Christmas Eve I planned; that night I prayed to God, "Thank you for the blessings of all my children and please help heal Chuck because we need him."

The next afternoon while I was visiting Chuck the doctor came in and said there was some pretty bad bruising and he would have a permanent numbness in his hip. The hip may bother him later on in life. They planned to get him up today and he can return home to rest and exercise. With a week off, we continued to celebrate Christmas. The kids had purchased a gift for me in town by themselves while Chuck was at the barber shop. They told me that everyone in the store knew that I had become the town's childcare director. The shop clerks thought they were very special to buy their Mom a gift. The kids said they did not have enough money to pay for the gift they chose. The clerks eagerly pitched in and not only completed paying for it but gift wrapped it. I was thrilled to unwrap a lovely light pink embroider country apron! It was such a gift of love. I adored the Cavalier towns' people of North Dakota. The commander even came over to see if we needed anything. He also told us in the rush to leave, we left the tree lights on. He walked over and turned them off. One of the branches had started to burn. Miraculously he was able to prevent a disaster. It was certainly a memorable Christmas.

We were happy to see our tour in North Dakota come to an end. The commander left the site and the new commander expunged Chuck's military record. We were even more exuberant because we had orders back to Colorado.

Chapter 17

We traveled three long days back to Colorado. We all screamed in excitement when we saw our Rocky Mountains. We found a cute little house to rent and we effortlessly reunited with our friends. We knew then that Colorado had become our home and we would retire there.

I was blessed that Mr. Smith hired me back with his company. I loved working for him and all the kids were in school and Brooke and Brandon could even come after school as needed.

We truly enjoyed raising our family. The years passed too quickly. Teen years were certainly challenging and always are. We had to constantly take Rick's car away but it was great bargaining power to lead him to graduation. We almost kissed the ground he walked on when he graduated. Then, we were so proud when he joined the Navy. I couldn't stop crying when we put him on the plane for boot camp. He served on ship in the Middle East. He sent me a gift from each port they docked. Shortly after Rick's departure, Chuck retired from the Air Force. His retirement was delayed because of DESERT STORM. He would have gone to Saudi Arabia but because Rick was actively serving he got to remain in Colorado. It was such a relief when Chuck finally retired. We gave him a wonderful party at a local Italian restaurant surrounded by family and co-workers. He immediately found work with a government contractor. Ryan grew into his manhood. He was easy going with so many friends. His social life was fabulous.

We had a health crisis with Chuck, Ryan's senior year. We did a family bowling night and he came home in so much pain. The next morning we took him to the emergency room at the Air Force Academy. The doctors felt he needed immediate surgery. The decision to operate was not finalized until late that night. Ryan was my strength that night. He sat with me outside the operating room. The surgery was taken a lot longer than they predicated. The corridors were empty except for one African American janitor. The janitor worked his way closer and I recognized his smile. He was our janitor at the childcare center. He started friendly conversation, "Hi there Miss Marion." I was pleased to talk to a friendly diversion.

"You work here, too?"

"Yes Ma'am, I moonlight here. It is good pay. I need all I can earn with four kids. They just called me over here because they had a surgery go bad. It's a real mess in that operating room. Why are you here so late?"

Unknowingly, he had set off an alarm of terror deep within my soul. With a shaky voice I replied, "My husband is having emergency surgery."

"Oh Miss Marion I am so sorry. I do apologize for opening my big mouth. There are great doctors in there. They are going to fix him up. Now you let me know if I can do anything!" He quickly scurried away.

Ryan couldn't hold back the tears. "Mom I need Dad so I can graduate. I love him so much." With those words I could not refrain from crying. Ryan embraced me and became my strength. It was still another hour before the doctor came to talk with us.

"Mrs. Barnes we removed your husband's appendix and when we realized it was fine we had to do exploratory surgery. He had Diverticulitis. We had to remove part of his intestines that was infected but because the colon could not be cleaned out we had to put in a colostomy bag. Mind you, this is only temporary." The doctor left and said Chuck would be in recovery a little longer than we could see him on the surgery floor in his room. I was shocked that he had a colostomy. I thanked God that he was alive! I was not prepared for the long days that followed. Chuck had such anguish over having this bag on his body. It caused a deep depression that I could not seem to lure him out of. I felt relief when Mom flew out to assist me. I still had to work because Chuck was losing forty percent of his pay. Mom was the queen of positive thinking. Patiently, she purchased nine pairs of slippers until he found a pair that satisfied him. His depression was compounded when a young, blonde, attractive, military doctor prepared him for discharge and in front of me and Mom told Chuck he could have a normal sex life.

He was appalled at her indiscretion and embarrassed. Chuck eventually got back to work but his temperament was not the same. He came home one day with the most staggering disclosure.

"Marion I think I know why God did this to me. I had lunch with a man that I work with. I did not know that he too, has a colostomy. His is for life from cancer. I have found a new empathy for people with disabilities."

"Chuck you know God has a plan for all of us." I was thrilled with the better attitude facing his every day challenges.

Before this medical crisis, Ricky had returned home from the Navy and had gotten married. They gave birth to a beautiful baby boy: our first Grandson. The baby, Michael Ryan, was Chuck's pride and joy.

Chuck returned for a surgery to reconnect and do away with the colostomy bag. The surgery was unsuccessful. He returned to such a state of depression he would not even get up out of bed. I left in a panic and asked my daughter-in-law if I could take Michael Ryan to the hospital. She packed his diaper bag and stroller. I pushed him into his grandfather's room.

"Chuck this is your grandson and he needs his grandfather. He needs you to take him fishing and to baseball games. Right now he needs you to get out of that bed and show him off!" With that, Chuck started to cry but pulled himself out of bed. He took hold of the stroller and started to stroll down the hospital corridor saying, "I want him to call me Pops!"

Chuck's folks came to visit until his next surgery. It was a good diversion and helped make time go faster. There was a bit of turmoil. Chuck's fears of a permanent colostomy haunted him. He was working and trying to spend time with his folks. There was a definite lack of intimacy going on. He felt less of a man. I reminded him of how he loved me even with out a bellybutton. He insisted it was not the same. I had never thought of Chuck as a big gambling man but the morning of his surgery he informed me, "I am stopping to get gas on the way to the hospital. Then I am going to purchase a lottery ticket. If it's a loser I will not have the surgery!" I looked at him and just shook my head. He jumped into his truck and scratched his one and only ticket. He won five hundred dollars. The surgery went on as scheduled and was successful. Thank you God! In time, Chuck seemed like a new person. He showed empathy to those who were ill. He seemed to appreciate life and fish more. Ryan graduated with his Dad looking on.

Brooke and Brandon were only one grade apart in school. Brandon loved his music. He sang in the honor choir. One time they performed at the very elite Broadmoor Hotel. He was very handsome and quite tall. He was so attractive in his tux. He missed the bus to come home. After work we drove to the hotel to pick him up. While we were there he gave us the grand tour. We paid valet to park. Brandon even offered to pay. Chuck asked, "Where did you get the money from?" He boastfully replied, "People thought I was the person that carried luggage to the rooms. Anybody who asked I carried their suitcases to their room and they gave me money!" While Chuck and I laughed he projected, "I think I will work here one day."

Brooke loved acting. She performed in programs whenever possible. She was tall and beautiful. She dressed stylishly. I drew the line when it came to belly shirts.

"Brooke those boys in high school will not be able to concentrate if you are showing your bellybutton! Besides I don't have a bellybutton, and I don't need to see anyone else's to remind me of that!" I went to pick her and her friends up from school one day. Out the girls came wearing belly shirts, I was furious. They lifted up there shirts as they got into my mini van. Over their bellybuttons were band aids marking an "X." Their giggles were contagious. I said, unsuccessfully, at avoiding laughter, "That's not funny!" Brooke always smiled even when she was in pain and she always cleaned when she was mad at me. She was so bright that she finished high school early. I kept my promise to her and her biological mother. I gave her all the information I had on her birth family when she turned 17. Together, we located their mother.

I knew Brooke always worried about her mother, so I hoped then that maybe she would find peace. Unknowingly, when Brooke was married and pregnant with her first child, she had set up a visit with Michelle, and she had invited Brandon. She did not tell me as to not hurt me, even though I understood, even encouraged it. But, I wasn't quite ready for Brandon to have another mom yet. She was a truck driver and came to Garden of the Gods to meet them. Brandon confided in me before he left to go meet her and it was so hard for me to let him venture out. I felt as if my heart skipped beats the whole time they were gone. I knew it was the right thing to do but self doubt overcame me. Did I protect them enough? Did I love them enough? Did they know that any mistakes I made I did it out of love? The agony lasted until Brandon came through the front door and said, "She is a great mother, but she is not Mom!" He flashed his sweet smile and all the agony disappeared. I knew I would always be their mom.

In 1997, I was saddened by my father's death. He had diabetes and was on dialysis. He needed surgery to open a vein in his leg. Mom called and said the surgery was a success. Within a few hours I received a call that he was struck with a heart attack and that I needed to go home. The whole flight, my mind wandered as I reflected back to the previous year. I was just so thrilled that I flew the kids home with me that fall for his 66th birthday. Chuck had planned a weekend fishing trip and I was bored. He told me to do anything I wanted so I called my brother George and we found a ticket sale. He helped with a loan to purchase enough for all of us. The boys had to fly on separate planes. Ricky spent the night at our house and we went to the airport. Ricky was 24 and Ryan 21. We went to get in the car and I heard Ricky say, "I am riding shotgun." Ryan protested, "You always ride shot gun!" I had to interject, "The oldest rides in the front there and Ryan you ride in the front coming home! Now let's go boys." Brooke and Brandon started laughing and then we all shared a magical moment. We arrived in Boston about ten minutes apart. The boys waved us down. Ricky was proudly carrying a bottle of champagne. The stewardess loved that they were visiting their sick grandfather and did not want the boys to go empty handed! We retrieved our baggage and excitedly searched the terminal looking for my brother. We didn't find him. But we did find a man holding a sign that read "Barnes Family." The kids were exhilarated to discover that George had sent a limousine for us. It was an amazing weekend. Now it had become a treasured memory.

I had pencil and paper and decided to write about Dad as tears poured down my cheeks. Dad if you die I am going to miss your remarkable sense of humor. Remember you always sent me one dollar equal to my age on every birthday. That was the only thrill of being forty. When I opened the card it had a twenty dollar bill in it with a note. *Sorry Marion, we all depreciate by fifty percent after forty!* I will miss you playing the jitterbug on the piano. I will miss the unique packages you always sent me. It had things like whoopee cushions and fancy hot dog holders and *Woods Real-Estate* calendars and newsletters. I will miss you picking me up at the airport and telling me all the news. I will miss all the post cards you have sent me from all your day trips and vacations. I will miss you calling Mom *The Mummy*. I will miss you putting on your sunglasses so we didn't see you with tears.

There were so many magical memories. Before we knew it we were landing. The moment we landed I saw my brother George waiting in baggage claim. He would not have left Dad's side otherwise so I knew Dad had passed during flight. He opened his arms to embrace and we both cried. Chuck and Ryan flew in for the funeral. There were five hundred people attending his wake. I found strength from God to write his eulogy. I went back to Colorado with a peaceful heart.

Working hard always helped me get back on track. I was posting parent's payments to their account and I got so distracted with the work that I had worked into part of my lunch hour. I quickly jumped up from my chair and saw that it was stained with blood. I went home to shower and change. I panicked when I found a growth. I immediately called for a doctor's appointment at the Air Force Academy hospital. Chuck and I discussed how I need to take care of this quickly and I was prepared for surgery. I couldn't believe the doctor that examined me had trained at Children's Hospital in Boston. He was fascinated with my case history. He actually was a medical student and observed one of my surgeries as a child. He informed me that I had a prolapsed colon. He said it would retract back in as long as I did not lift anything. He said surgery was not recommended due to all my scar tissue. I left discouraged and angry with God.

This was not like me. I talked to myself on the drive home from the doctor's. "God, I have struggled to be healthy. I had all these surgeries! I don't need to be a freak now with a colon coming out!" In such turmoil, I continued to yell at Him, "How could you do this? I am so angry! Tell me why!" I had arrived at the commissary to pick up some groceries while I was on base. I usually smiled at people passing, but not today. I just purchased what I needed and headed to the cash register. There was a person in front of me. He was a tall, balding, handsome man. The stranger caught my eyes because he was the spitting image of my Uncle Tommy. I had such a profound respect for Uncle Tommy. He inspired everyone around him. Tommy always had a warm smile and never judged a soul. He was also an amazing speaker. He worked in Washington D.C. with the health education and welfare department for many years. When the man behind the counter turned around he had a huge growth on the side of his neck. It appeared to be a goiter. Still in my cantankerous mood, I quickly checked out. I headed to the base gas station. There, the same man was in front of me pumping his gas. I waited my turn. It was odd. I couldn't see the growth on the side of his neck. When the man completed pumping his gas, he looked straight at me. There was a huge growth right on his face. It was so big that I gasped. I was covered with goose bumps because of a haze or rather a glow around him. I turned away so as not to stare. When I looked back in a matter of seconds he had disappeared. I was eager to go home. I drove out of the Academy. The road leaving the shopping complex is so peaceful. I never realized how tall the pine trees were. As the sun broke through the clouds, I was suddenly filled with peace. "God," I cried out, "I get it! I could have growths on my face or be stricken with things far more serious! I am so sorry for doubting you! Thank you for answering my questions!" My soul found a much needed peacefulness. From that point on, I believed Uncle Tommy, who died an agonizing death from nerve cancer, was my guardian angel. I found my smile and was ready for my new challenge, gracefully.

Work was a real challenge, directing a childcare center and not being able to lift was almost impossible. I had the most outstanding staff ever; they would ask me to cover their classroom while they unloaded food orders and teaching supplies. I just did not have the temperament to watch others and not help. I loved the team we had put together. We all thought alike. We didn't just take care of the child but the whole family. I had my own philosophy of childcare. Childcare should be a home away from home. While curriculum was important, we never passed on a teachable moment. Our center was warm and loving. We nurtured families from diverse backgrounds and special needs children. The staff always felt that we had created our own little ministry. We put on elaborate graduation and holiday performances with rented chairs and stages. If a child did not have holiday clothes the staff provided them. With the state requiring more certification in classes for medication, CPR, blood pathogens, continuing education, and disaster readiness exhausted all of us. Unlike other businesses, you could not take a day off without someone to care for the children. We had to keep in ratio of teachers per children. There were times when we worked extended hours to make this happen. We all loved our work and did it. With all the new requirements, I am pleased to report that we did not have a big turnover; however, the days of hiring a grandmother because of her love of children were over. The days of carefree playing in the park were gone. The days of spontaneously hugging or kissing a child on the forehead were gone. We live in fear of being misjudged or sued. We were able to overcome these fears and provide the best quality childcare possible. All of us would seriously discuss our deep concerns for the future of childcare. The cost of childcare had to drastically increase to meet these new regulations. We could not help but wonder how many children were being left alone or left in unsafe settings because of the cost. Each day we faced new circumstances in this evolving career. We never forgot and constantly applied the most important rule: To love the way God loves us, love the children and watch them bloom.

My own children were certainly blooming. Brandon was in his senior year and in love. His girlfriend's mother was deaf. We were so proud of him when he became completely fluent in sign language. Brooke had joined the Air Force. It was a short lived career. She chose to get out after she took a fall that damaged her ankle. But, we also knew what a good actress she was, too. She came home with hilarious stories like how her nail polish was not okay and how they called her "Red" instead of Brooke. She even asked Chuck, "Could you believe they yelled at me when I was eating?" We laughed so hard. We all agreed the military life was not for Brooke. Unfortunately, we had already turned her room into an office. But, shortly after her return she did enrolled in college. We knew that was where she belonged.

Ryan had married a lovely girl from his college. She had two adorable little boys from a previous marriage. Ricky's wife had her precious daughter, Lacey, come live with them. Our family grew by leaps and bounds.

It was an amazing family celebration when Brandon graduated. Both our families came to celebrate. Chuck's dad gave Brandon a bible for a graduation gift. Brandon was more touched that Grandpa Barnes put his name in the Barnes' family bible. Chuck's dad, Joseph, had to leave the celebration early and go back to Florida. He told us he just wasn't feeling well and felt he needed to go home and rest.

Chapter 17

One gorgeous day I looked out my bedroom window. I was mesmerized by the cloud formation. The clouds slowly moved and formed a perfect cross. An ominous feeling came over me. I knew something was about to happen. That was the beginning of my journey with Joseph. Later in the evening we got the call from Chuck's family. His father had become so ill they sent him to a larger hospital in Dothan, Alabama. He was diagnosed with terminal lung cancer. He requested for us to stay put. They gave him five years to live with chemotherapy. We cried and assured ourselves that he would survive.

Before the week was over, Joseph had a reaction to the chemo. They did not think he would make it through the night. We got on the first flight we could find. Chuck's brother, Dennis, picked us up at the airport. Then, we drove with him from Atlanta to Dothan.

Chuck's hands were trembling as we entered the intensive care unit. We were taken back from the strange odor in the room. Joseph was happy to see us. He was surprisingly alert. Medical personnel told us that the next twenty four hours were critical but Joseph pulled through the night. It gave me such pleasure to see Chuck and his dad have some quality time together. The doctor reassured us that he still had three to five good years left. With Joseph in stable condition, we were able to return home. I relived my own father dying as my plane landed.

In a short three weeks later, we were called back saying that his dad became ill with E. coli and was on his death bed. This was too much of a financial burden to pick up and fly again so we drove. Joseph chose to go to the local hospital close to his church friends and family. Once again, we rushed to the hospital.

We quietly entered the hospital room and Joseph opened his eyes and looked up at Chuck. "Well hi there Charles you came back."

Chuck responded, "I sure did. I heard you are not doing so well. Is there anything I can do for you?"

"Charles, I sure would love some chicken nuggets. Do you reckon you can run to McDonalds and get me some?"

Chuck was taken by surprise by his request. "Sure Dad that is the least I can do."

Chuck and I went to McDonalds. "Chuck are you sure he is on his death bed?"

"Marion I am very confused. Dennis flew in from New York and he is concerned too."

"Well, we can't afford to come to give the family moral support each time he has a set back or complications."

"Denis said the same thing. Maybe we just need to be moral support for Mom."

"She looks so worn out. They have been married for more than fifty years." We returned with the chicken nuggets. Chuck's dad relished the smell of them. He only took baby bites and we noticed how difficult it was for him to swallow. He couldn't finish them. We all went back to the house, which seemed longer than eleven miles away. Chuck's Mom said she needed to talk to all of us before we retired for the night.

She spoke with authority. "I am glad you are all here. The doctor says there is not much time. I am exhausted and I need your help. I am making a schedule of times for all of you to be at the hospital. We don't all need to be there together at this time. If you are not at the hospital you can prepare dinner or do some of the chores." In unison, we all agreed and somberly went to bed.

The next day I was to be at the hospital at eleven in the morning to relieve Yvonne, my mother-in-law. I arrived a little early so I tip-toed into the room, unnoticed. I encountered the most romantic moment I had ever seen. Joseph motioned for Yvonne to come over to his bed.

"Yvonne, help me stand up. I want to hold you and kiss you like a man one last time while I still can." Joseph got a steady foot and he adjusted his hospital gown and wrapped his arms around her and kissed her passionately. I had to leave the room so no one could see my tears.

Joseph had fallen into a deep sleep before Yvonne left. He had a continuing flow of visitors. I walked in the hall to greet each one and thank them for visiting. Most did not know me so I devotedly introduced myself. Unexpectedly, I was taken aback from what I saw and felt. Every hand I reached out to shake caused a warm, burning sensation that bled into my hand and when I looked up at their faces they were surrounded by a celestial aura. These humble, Godly people all shared acts of kind deeds or financial assistance they had received from Joseph. He performed simple little deeds like driving the senior Sunday school bus even though he was a senior himself. He repaired roofs, or fixed broken equipment and laid brick. He had done all these deeds without boasting. I could not perceive at this time why God allowed me to really see these people. I was uncertain of why God had chosen to reveal this to me. I did know that I, too, wanted to have that celestial aura around me someday.

The following evening we all gathered during visiting hours in Joseph's room. His breathing had started to become laborious. He was resting, so I talked quietly with my sister-in-law, Brenda. Glancing out the window, I could see the sun had set and it was getting dark. Abruptly, I was startled by an amazing bolt of white light that penetrated through the window and right inside of me. In the depths of my soul, I felt a euphoric sensation. This sensation felt like goose bumps that one receives from doing a wonderful deed but multiplied by a billion times. I sat in awe of this amazing moment and froze in time. I was slowly aroused only to contemplate the question in my mind: Had Joseph died? My sister in law asked me, "Marion, are you okay? You seemed to have this blank look on your face."

Softly, I asked her, "Did you see the light?"

"Yes I did see a flash of light and you got a blank look."

We both looked over at Joseph. I actually thought he had died. I was astonished when Joseph had opened his eyes.

He called out directly to me, "Marion wasn't my journey beautiful?" He had such a peaceful smile on his face.

"Yes, Dad it was amazing."

"I wanted to share it with you."

I was totally perplexed by all these experiences. I did not have a moment to analyze any of these wonders. Joseph once again appeared full of life as he teased me.

"Marion I knew you thought I was dead or dying but it was a Catholic Angel. The Baptist one will come later!" We all laughed and relished his sense of humor no one else realized that we had shared a majestic moment. Joseph died the following night grasping for air but he died with such grace and dignity.

I was so busy that I could not find time or a quiet moment to contemplate all that had happened. Yvonne did what she had to do but was obviously exhausted and still in shock.

She was trying to reason why God took Joseph first. She had battled cancer and won three times. Her belief was: God took Joseph now so her son Don could move in and take care of her. Don only stuck his head in to check on his father. He was unable to watch his agony. Don had just lost his wife Pat, five months prior. She had a very long struggle with lung cancer that continued to spread all over her body with horrific pain and blindness at the end. Yvonne's reasoning did make sense. I think God had a different plan. Before the funeral, Don invited me and his brothers out to lunch. We arrived early and Don walked in with a lively woman at his side. She was slender with long dark hair and loved to laugh. Don was quite taken with her. It was so pleasing to see him happy. He pulled me aside and asked, "Marion, do you think it is okay for me to take her to Dad's funeral."

I knew he needed strength at the time more than ever and replied, "Absolutely!"

I then took on the task of preparing his mother. I needed to let her know that Don was ready to move on. When I explained it to her, she seemed to accept it gracefully.

The funeral was simple and spiritual. Chuck's sister had the hardest time of all. She was hysterical before the services. We could all feel her heartache. No one had the words to soothe her. She was after all, being the only girl, a daddy's girl. After we returned home she told us she found peace when she saw her dad sitting on the front porch in the rocking chair.

I finally had found time to have quiet time with God. I sat on my porch looking up at the mountains and started to ponder over all the events that took place with Joseph's death. Then, slowly it was all clear. I was given the gift of peace. Because of all my birth defects I always feared dying. By revealing the beauty of death, God raked the fear out of my soul. I pondered the damage that fear can do to one's soul. Then I realized, fearing death, meant fearing living and with fear of failure how can one possibly succeed? I also feared aging! I didn't want wrinkles. I am sure Moses looked like a prune but I know what he accomplished with his life.

I grasped that the gift of my life was so precious and not to be wasted. I guess if we cannot figure it out we just turn it over to God. I made the choice to live my life zestfully. I want my life to always be filled with love and laughter. Since I had already learned to embrace peace, I also wanted to never forget how to be able to show compassion, empathy, and strength. I also realized that I want to live without fear so I can be an achiever. I promised God I would share my new knowledge. I knew some would think I was hallucinating or imagined some of it but I was fearless of the truth.

I tried to be fearless as all my children's marriages as they fell apart. Chuck and I tried to be supportive. Those turbulent times played havoc with relationships. I was seriously seeking an answer to our despair. Four children; four divorces, and torn families were the root of all this despair. My health had me realize with much sorrow, I needed to retire as well. I had such a passion for my work. Part-time would be okay but the company had no part-time director positions. I offered to step down and teach but I had supervised for so long they felt it would not have worked out. Mr. Smith gave me a wonderful retirement party in his distinguished home, a home that Chuck, in his short, part-time career of being a realtor, had sold him. The sale of his previous home and new home allowed us to be financially more secure to make the transition into retirement. Having my first summer off in twenty years was like an island vacation. Our new home had parks and access to our community pool. Once all the grandchildren went back to school the after glow of retirement wore off. Chuck was working for a government contract in Cheyenne Mountain. He did not like his position at all. In order to find a way out he went back to college. The family was so proud of him when he achieved his goal. He attained another position for less pay. In order for us to manage financially, I had started consulting for a local childcare center. It filled in my empty gaps of time. I felt working six hours a day would be within my physical limitations. We still had major concerns with our children's lives. Chuck shared these concerns with his mother and she insisted we read Rick Warren's book *Purpose of Driven Life*. While Chuck and I had both attended Christian colleges, we both had a mental block about reading this book.

Chapter 18

Our lives stayed so busy. We took time out to travel for my brother's birthday in December. It was the holiday season and New England is so festive. I spent time with all my siblings. I especially wanted to see a dear family friend, a beautiful Christian woman whose life was full of many good deeds. I left a small, anonymous gift for her under the tree. We went forth on our vacation and celebrated George's fiftieth birthday. George and I are *Irish Twins*, born in the same year. So, he honored me with a cake also. Exhausted by all our activities, we were ready to depart for the airport. In the driveway of Mom's house, walked that special family friend and with her she carried a little brown gift bag. We went outside to give her a hug. And she told us how she discovered the gift was from us, "You guys, I appreciate your gift under the tree." Her voice was so sweet.

I replied, "It's not much!"

She then presented us with her gift bag. "Here is a little something for your flight home to read."

"Thank you. You didn't need to do that! We love you but we have to get going to the airport." We loaded the car for our departure and bid farewell to the whole gang that had gathered to see us off.

Once on the plane, we pulled out the book. It was *The Purpose Driven Life*.

We both felt God had intended for us to read this book. I could not put it down. Then, I began reading it aloud to Chuck. He actually listened attentively. We even had an intriguing discussion about it. Once completed, we had established a mission. The book revealed all Rick Warren's beliefs of pursuing a purposeful life. In our life we practiced most of what he recommended: all except one. We did not belong to a church together. Actually, Chuck had stopped going to church. Who says a Catholic and Protestant can't find a church? So, our mission was to find a church.

At a real estate Christmas party I had a conversation with a young mother over a social glass of wine. I shared my mission with her and she proudly described the joy she had found in her church, Woodmen Valley Chapel. She eagerly invited us to attend.

We did attend and some other churches too. We fell in love with the Woodmen mission and their vision of growth. It was a much larger church than we were seeking but we wanted to make it our own, much like the words of John f. Kennedy and my wonderful cousin Diane: It's not what your church can offer you but what you can offer a church. It also brought me such peace. My Catholicism was there for me but took Chuck away from his church. With all my health issues, I felt Chuck needed a church to help guide him through what ever the future might hold. I found so much joy in giving him back to God. God was just patiently waiting for him to return to his house: our new church. He joined the men's ministry and gave of himself generously. I knew God was pleased to have him back.

Puzzle like pieces seemed to fall into place. All the children formed new healthy strong relationships. Our son Ryan's divorced wife, Lori, came to Church and became a member. She brought with her our granddaughters. They were both baptized there. They assisted me in the children's ministry. Ryan and Lori even remarried in the church. Brooke fell in love with a wonderful, spiritual, retired NFL player. They married in the church and their baby girl was christened there. Our daughter was baptized there. Brandon and his girlfriend began attending. Ricky remarried formed a strong relationship.

The center I was consulting became far more than I had anticipated. The owner developed terminal cancer. I worked, cooking and tried to keep the staff from knowing the center may close. A much bigger challenge was the owner's cynicism about God. I spent hours talking to her and hoping she could find peace in her death. She desperately believed God could not forgive her for all her sins. She said there were no such thing as free choice and forgiveness. When she died, I did not know if she was a believer. I prayed the hours I talked with her helped her to believe.

I just hope that when my time comes I want to be ready and go peacefully. I want to die with dignity and grace. I know I will be filled with and the glory of God and belief in the savior Jesus Christ so my journey would be complete.

The consulting job was physically draining. I decided to go to a childcare center and teach their private kindergarten program. I enjoyed each day the first year. The second year, ownership changed. Teachers were required do head counts every fifteen minutes. Teachers were required to clean bathrooms and mop floors. So many distractions from the children made teaching less enjoyable and took so much time away from learning. These last three years were too much physical hardship on my body, even just working part-time. I had no choice except to permanently retire.

Chapter 19

There are some wonderful things about retirement. Every fall I would fly, and still do to Cape Cod. I join Mom and my sisters for a week vacation. Mom has a time share in Falmouth, Massachusetts on the Cape. It is so close to the beach. We do everything from shopping, to long walks around the beach. We find wonderful restaurants to eat, preferably with ocean views. The shopping is the greatest. Many shops start clearance sales before they close for the winter. Mom often shares with us memories of the activities that she and Dad did on the Cape. We know this brings her great joy. Each year we find a new adventure, like a boat ride to Martha's Vineyard or a trip to Hyannis Port. I must say my favorite adventure was whale watching. The whales amazed me with their massive beauty and gentleness. They traveled with their calves and their fins shined with a florescent aquamarine glow. We have made so many memories there. When my lovely nieces would join us for a weekend we giggled and laughed and ate too much. I loved how once they gave me a head to toe make over to go back home to their Uncle Chuck. I had a polka dotted blouse and my hair was straightened. It was great for my ego. After that trip Chuck was convinced that I was having too much fun and he planned to join me the following year.

That September we took our annual trip to the mountains to see the golden Aspen trees before we departed for the trip to the Cape. I envisioned all the things I wanted to experience with Chuck on our vacation. Chuck and I were talking about the joy of being able to see the Aspens and the brilliant New England foliage in the same month. Chuck went down stairs to bring our luggage up from the storage room so we could air it out before we packed them. The phone rang and it was Mom.

"Marion, your brother Kenny won't be able to pick you up at the airport. I know he always does but this time John will come get you." Then she started to cry.

"Mom, what is wrong."

"Remember I told you Kenny was so constipated he went to the emergency room?"

"Yes."

"They ran tests and discovered he has colon cancer." I cried with her. Then, I realized I needed to be comforting her. "They have come so far with all kinds of treatments. I will be there in a couple of days."

The enthusiasm over our planned trip had changed. By the time we had arrived, Kenny was diagnosed with advanced stages of a fast growing cancer. The course of action was chemotherapy. Chuck and I were both so happy that God allowed us this time with family. We knew Kenny had a tough road ahead of him. He could have been placed in a hospice but Mom would not do that. Since Dad's death, Kenny took wonderful care of her. He took her to doctor appointments and carried in her groceries. Kenny was a carpenter and he built her a huge walk in closet for her bedroom. Every morning he walked to Dunkin Donuts and bought her fresh coffee. He was a simple man with a big heart. He wore his dirty blonde hair long and clean braided down his back. He was available to help anyone in need. Kenny talked slowly. You would think he had a lower I.Q., but that was never the case. We were all shocked when he passed his test for his real-estate license the first time. Mom prepared her living room for Kenny's hospital bed and special needs. She purchased memory foam for the bed so he would be comfortable. She intended, with her strong will, to nurture him back to good health. He was experiencing back pain in the hospital. We were there to welcome him home from the hospital. He appeared to look and act like himself. He took charge and planned to have his beard and hair cut short to prepare for his hair loss. Chuck and I left to stay at a hotel. The second day we went to check on him and he had walked to buy me a hot cup of tea and even helped me up Mom's front porch. His appearance with the short hair shocked us. He looked more fragile and older with more gray hair showing. His eagerness to help me touched my heart. He kept apologizing for not being able to pick me up. Dad always picked me up and Kenny took that job over with pride. Our day with him was beautiful. Mom washed a bowl of grapes for a snack. Chuck started eating them and Kenny joined him saying, "Chuck, these grapes are good. I have never eaten grapes before. I need to start eating more like Mom." Mom added, "Yes you should. Grapes are a great antioxidant!" Kenny said, "I plan on eating healthy and quitting smoking. I am going to beat this disease."

Later that afternoon Ken answered the office door attached off of Mom's kitchen. It was a neighbor needing Mom's notary services. After she left, Kenny proceeded to have an amazing conversation with me. "The lady at the door is one of the neighbors. Her car broke down in the snow and I helped her. I have tried to help all the neighbors. I have been thinking about all the good deeds I have done in my life."

"Kenny I know God knows all the good you have done. I hope you believe." He nodded his head yes and tears swelled in his eyes. "Our conversation was interrupted with a phone call from my sister Ruth. "Marion, Beth reserved a limo for Kenny to attend John's and Jill's thirtieth wedding party tomorrow night. That way he can ride in comfort. It's a surprise so don't tell him. Beth said she would be honored if you joined them in the limo." "Awe! That would be wonderful!" I said. Beth, was Kenny's girlfriend.

The next evening we were all at mom's before the limo arrived. Kenny called Beth into the family room saying he needed to talk to her. Beth proceeded to the back room and all of a sudden we heard a scream of joy. She was crying and laughing at the same time. On her finger was a diamond ring. Kenny informed her it was a forever ring. Kenny looked out on the porch and asked, "Who is the limo for?" Beth squealed in a high pitched voice, "I hired it for us Kenny! You said that John ruined your second birthday party by being born on your birthday and you knew it would ruin his anniversary party just by showing up . . . because you said everybody presumes you are on your death bed! Let's go in style and show them you are full of life." We all loaded into the stretch limo and headed for the party. Beth was still crying and enjoying every moment with Kenny.

I couldn't help but remember Kenny and Beth's history. They dated in high school. Kenny had the biggest crush on her. Beth's father had forbidden her from dating him because he had a truck. Beth and Kenny went their separate ways. Beth's sister stopped one day at Mom's home office and asked all about the Woods' boys, Kenny in particular. When Beth found out Kenny was at home with Mom she called and talked to him. In their forties, they fell in love all over again.

We arrived at the anniversary party. We wanted Kenny and Beth to enter last. As we expected, Kenny was the center of attention. He became surrounded by all our family, receiving joyous hugs and well wishes.

I approached John and Jill and said, "I know Kenny's presence has put your celebration in a different light."

John said with tears of joy, "I am honored to share our life celebration of thirty years with my brother and celebrate his life also! We are officially calling our party a celebration of life!" John and his beautiful wife, Jill, embraced me. My brother George and his band performed for the event. It was a heart wrenching evening. The band's lead singer Juan had just lost his precious wife to cancer. George's amazing wife, Carol, had just lost her brother to cancer. The band called Kenny and John on stage to join them. We all knew John could sing but were we shocked to hear Kenny burst out in song. Then, John and Kenny started to play air guitar. In amazement, the whole audience joined in playing air guitar. Kenny left the stage saying that was something he always wanted to do but couldn't gather enough courage. How wonderful that he had that opportunity. With the musical talent in our family it was hard not to be intimidated to sing or perform. The magic of the night did not stop there. We took beautiful pictures with Mom. We were all here together and I could feel God's presence among us. The lead singer Juan burst into a song, *"How Far is Heaven."* We all made a circle of life and surrounded Kenny. There was not a dry eye in the room. Juan's God given voice touched all our hearts. Juan uses his gift for benefits and even to support the homeless shelters. George's amazing drum solo played next followed by our family celebration song, *"We are Family."* Kenny informed us it was the best party of his life.

We all escaped for a weekend to the Cape. Ruth and I developed pictures to savor our memories of this week. We all believed Mom would help the doctors heal Kenny. But, he only lived about a month after his diagnosis. Mom called me to come home she did not think he would make it through the weekend. Patty said Kenny was in terrible pain causing Mom deep agony. All my siblings and their spouses stayed all night at the hospital. Patty said she witnessed the most amazing love between a mother and child. Mom stood up and said, "I can't bear this anymore." Mom went to Kenny's bedside. She proceeded to rub his back and whisper. "Kenny I know you are a fighter but its okay to go into the light. Just go into the light." Kenny totally relaxed and took his last breath.

My family was honored to have several hundred people attend Kenny's wake. I had to rest on a chair in the receiving line. The funeral parlor had a website where people blogged on Kenny's page. We were touched by special memories from so many entries. Kenny moonlighted as a bouncer at a pub called Abbey Road. Years ago, in Kenny's youth, he had a DUI. After that, he made up his mind never to drink alcohol again. The pub became a place where he could engage with others and make a difference. Reading the blogs of how he made sure people got home safely and kept the peace made me reflect on my own son Ricky. Ricky wanted to be a bartender but always bar backed or cooked in a local pub. He lacked confidence. He was also experiencing marital problems. One late afternoon he came over and asked if he could move back home.

He could not fix his marriage. He had already experienced one broken marriage. A storm was lingering over the city. We were all sitting in our home office when a golden hue shined through the window. We went out on the porch and saw these large cumulous clouds ascending in front of our home. Rick and Chuck ran out into the street to get a closer look. Rick came running back into the house saying, "Mom I need a camera I saw Jesus." He ran back into the street and took several pictures. Tears were streaming down his face. Ricky was not spiritual. He believed everything could be explained by science. He came in with the camera and Chuck downloaded the pictures on to the computer. Sure enough we all saw Jesus in all the pictures. Rick slid to his knees and out loud said, "Thank you God." He stood up and said, "Thanks Mom and Dad I know what I need to do. I am going home and saving my marriage." Not only was he able to save his marriage, he became a bartender and the picture of Jesus sits behind his bar. Our Church's lead pastor reeled me into our church when he opened a sermon with the song "*I Love this Bar.*" The pastor said Churches needed to be more like bars. In bars, people engage with each other helping them through everyday life experiences. They celebrate birthdays, births, marriages and even deaths. They form their own community. Kenny made part of his legacy at his pub. He will be forever remembered by all of us who loved him.

Chapter 20

During my decision on early retirement, Chuck had earned two promotions so financially we would be okay; but, he encouraged me to file for disability.

"Marion you are disabled and have been your whole life. I know you just want to be normal but you are not. You may need that extra medical care one day."

"Chuck it is embarrassing to tell everyone what is physically wrong with me. Besides, I looked online and you have to get medical exams and a million forms."

He then demanded, "Well if you are going to file and see their doctors you are going to get checked again to see if there is something to help you or help with the pain."

I agreed to go to the doctors once again. I was sent to a specialist in Denver. Once again the diagnosis was that everything at that time was inoperable. The doctors feared making things worse since there were no road maps of my previous surgeries. I had massive amounts of scar tissue. They also were concerned that I might have cancer. Fortunately, the biopsy was negative. I was pleased with my present condition thinking it could have been worse, like cancer.

Realizing that I could not work again and my lifestyle had to alter, I reluctantly filed for disability with Social Security. It was quite a tedious process. I filled out paper work online. I answered questions like: Do you have a dog? How do you care for your dog? There were phone interviews. I had to collect all my doctors' visits, surgeries, procedures and diagnosis. People told me I needed a lawyer but I was stubborn and did it on my own. I figured if I did not receive this benefit I wasn't deserving of it. The state sent me for x-rays and routine test. I felt like a criminal. I was checked and double checked to prove my identity. I was told it was to prevent fraud. All I could think was who would actually *want* to be labeled as disabled? I was granted my disability the first time. My reaction astonished me. I did not expect to feel relieved, but I did. It gave me a little financial security and extra medical insurance. Also, I was relieved that I would not be a burden to my husband.

My husband became my strength the following year. I could not stand in one place longer than five minutes without excruciating pain. I could not sit long with out pain. The agony had doubled in the last year after receiving my disability. The worst was the constant bleeding. I accepted everything gracefully. I still volunteered at the hospital and at the church to do storytelling. At the hospital, I tried working in outpatient surgery but it was to painful pushing the wheelchairs. I ended up volunteering at the gift shop. I left ready to go home and lay down but while I was there I felt alive being able to contribute. I made a dear friend, Donna. I retired much too young so most of my friends still worked. Donna was my height with a tiny frame and soft blonde hair. She shared her strong spirituality with me and we instantly became close friends. The people we met there often shared their joys and sorrows with us while visiting the shop. A woman with soft gray hair came in walking slowly as if she was very uncomfortable. I began to have a conversation with her.

"Can I help you find anything?"

She replied, "I am just looking thank you."

She started to look at our display of willow tree angels. I approached her and stated, "Aren't they lovely? I have a small collection of them myself."

The sweet lady responded. "They sure are. I am just so happy to be out and about. I am moving slowly because I had colon surgery a few weeks ago."

This of course intrigued me. "You are getting around great. Is everything all repaired now?" She moved a little closer and lowered her voice as she said "My colon prolapsed and I was even losing control. I thought I had cancer. It just bled and bled. I had gotten to the point where I didn't want to go anywhere."

I comfortably poured out my own condition to her. "I have a prolapsed colon too. It's miserable! The doctors told me there was nothing that could be done."

She responded eagerly, "You need to go see my doctor in Parker, Colorado. My primary sent me to him. He keeps up with all the new procedures. Here let me give you his name." She continued, "It is Dr. John Sun. If he can't help you, no one can."

I quickly wrote down the information she gave me. I turned around to thank her and she was gone but she left me with a spark of hope. I went home and immediately called Chuck. "Honey, I met this wonderful lady who just had surgery for her prolapsed colon. She gave me the doctor's name and he is in Parker, Colorado." Before he could reply, I eagerly continued, "He is a specialist. I was put on Medicare so I don't need a referral. I am so excited but I shouldn't get my hopes up. He may not take our insurance. I know I am unique and more complicated with all my past surgeries."

Chuck replied, "Marion you have nothing to lose I will support you in what ever you decide to do. Go ahead and call for an appointment."

I hung up the phone and called information for Dr. Sun's number and immediately called him. His receptionist answered the phone.

"May I help you?"

"I sure hope so. I would like to make an appointment with Dr. Sun."

I explained my condition and gave her my insurance information. My heart skipped a beat with excitement when she said the doctor could see me in two weeks. She completed our conversation like my little, gray-headed, sweet angel, "If he can't help you no one can. He has many happy patients from all over."

I shared my great news with Chuck and Donna. I kept catching myself getting too excited and asking myself who gets excited about seeing a colon doctor?

Two weeks went quickly. Chuck took off early and drove me to the hospital. We loved the quaint town of Parker right outside of Denver. The town is small and quite modern. We located the hospital easily. My stomach was turning from nerves as we entered the doctor's office. It was a small office decorated in a Far East décor. I signed in for the appointment next to a toilet shaped candle. The pens sat in a mug decorated with animal bottoms! Chuck had picked up a photo album that sat on the coffee table. He shared the contents with me. First, there were pictures labeled of the Dr.'s sons, they read, #1 Sun and #2 Sun, with a play on the word *son*! The quiet office filled with our laughter. Then we viewed pictures of Dr. Sun performing surgeries on mission trips around the world. My nerves calmed down and I knew I was in good hands. I knew God sent me here. Dr. Sun scheduled many tests to help make a plan to operate. He wanted to make a road map of all my past surgeries but I had wires in me preventing an MRI from being performed. He devised a plan and scheduled it for the first week in September. At that point, I was ready to tell Mom. She was thrilled, but preferred me to have surgeries in Boston. I told her she did not need to attend. "Marion, nothing will keep me away. I will be there until you are healed!" Naturally, she would be there; although she was experiencing her own trouble with her feet from complications from diabetes. Chuck picked up Mom from the Denver airport and they both were at my side for the surgery. Amazingly enough, I was quite relaxed. We entered pre-op and outside of my cubical, hung the most amazing picture. The title read: *Chief of the Medical Staff; By Nathan Greene.* Jesus rested his hands on surgeons during an operation. It brought tears to Mom's and Chuck's eyes.

Mom was determined to find a copy of the painting. My surgery had complications and I ended up in intensive care. The doctor removed a four centimeter pro-lapse. I was able to recover and go home. I experienced apprehension concerning the return of the pro-lapse. I started to heal and miraculous things came about. I could walk without feeling that horrible pain and pressure. There was no bleeding. My ankle swelling decreased.

I lost thirty pounds. I was taken off of blood pressure medicine and two other medications. I could function with a zestful energy: I know I still can not lift and my hip can pop out and I have back pain. My left leg doesn't lift all the time but I can dance even in pain. That pain is manageable. God must still need me here.

I thank him every day for all my blessings. I want everyday to count. I am thankful for the beautiful people that have enriched my life.

My adult life I spent journaling and writing short stories. I promised God that if I survived my last surgery that I would finish all my stories and complete my book. I reflected on my promise on this glorious Colorado morning. The sun flickered on my face coming through my oblong stained glass hanging over the window above my fireplace. I walked through the front room and opened the white glass French doors into the office. I pulled down my thesaurus and dictionary and placed it next to the computer and began to write my life story. I wanted a book that would inspire those with handicaps to become achievers, to reach out and find God. Then, readers will discover: With God all things are possible. We need to let go of the anger caused by being different. We are going to sin like everyone else, forgive yourself put it behind you and move forward. Work hard and find a place you can fit and begin to achieve. My vision of God is that he sits in heaven putting together our life puzzle. Eventually, all the pieces come together. We should get rid of any fears holding us back. Most importantly, learn to forgive and love with all our hearts. Before my surgery, I peacefully wrote letters to all my children in case God did not want me on Earth any longer. I even prepared my funeral service. What I did not tell anyone was that Dr. Sun said he could make me a bellybutton. My reply was, "No thank you, my life couldn't be any better with a bellybutton!"

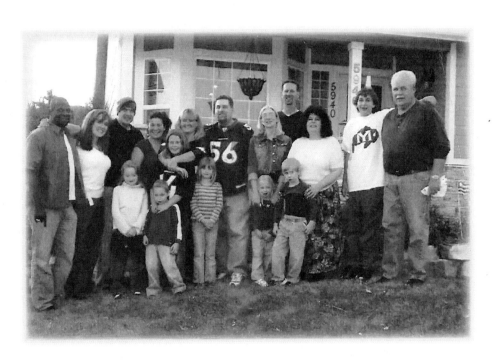